"I'm

Sorry,

It's Pancreatic Cancer"

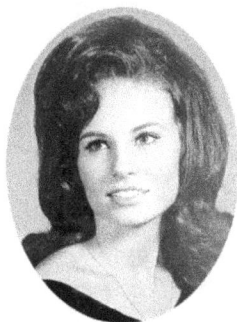

"I'm

Sorry,

It's Pancreatic Cancer"

Gary Doyen

Jacket and interior design by The Book Cover Whisperer:
ProfessionalBookCoverDesign.com

ISBN: 978-0-578-56074-8 Paperback
ISBN: 978-0-578-56079-3 eBook

Printed in the U.S.A.

FIRST EDITION

This work is dedicated to the persons who have suffered or are now suffering with pancreatic cancer and those who love and care for them. This book is simply one of your stories.

Contents

Acknowledgements

For a first-time attempt at becoming a published author, it takes more than those long hours, days, weeks, and months of writing alone to bring a work to fruition. There are not enough words to express my gratitude to my brother, Mick Doyen. He took second drafts with notes and corrections attached and was able to decipher enough to get the manuscript neatly typed in the computer. In addition, with his practice as an English teacher for forty years, he edited each page relentlessly. Thank you, Mick.

My daughter, Sarah, also an accomplished English teacher, diligently went over the final edition, editing and getting it into a "Word document." Thank you, Sarah.

To Christopher Miller, a dear and very knowledgeable friend, for lending me valuable techniques concerning the process, while at the same time, telling me the truths of the difficult task at hand. Thank you, Chris.

And lastly to my daughter, Andrea, who graciously shared her own journals for me to use. They were priceless! Thank you, Andrea.

Introduction

Here I sit looking throughout this room trying to imagine myself back in time to see the beige, leather sofa where my wife, Dava, would lie with her pillow and blanket. I envision her beautiful, brown reddish hair, now a thinning gray color. Her eyes are closed, giving her a silent reprieve from the constant pain emanating from the cancer cells attacking her pancreas and liver. Every room in the house still exudes her creative and decorative touch; the half curtains on the living room windows and the framed painting of a small house with Dava's own written inscription, "Bless this Home with Love and Daughters" still adorn our home.

Sometimes my heart aches, wondering if Dava and I did everything that was possible. Was there something we didn't know about and missed, and did we attempt to do the supernatural? I really don't know, but my total focus was to have her with me as long as she was able to withstand the torture and suffering and to preserve her willingness to fight the cancer. Never have I witnessed courage in such a tolerant and unselfish way. I can now more fully understand the harsh truth in this excerpt from Robert

Frost's "Home Burial" :

> "... The nearest friends can go
> With anyone to death, comes so far short
> They might as well not try to go at all.
> No, from the time one is sick to death,
> One is alone, and he dies more alone.
> Friends make pretense of following to the grave,
> But before one is in it, their minds are turned
> And making the best of their way back to life.
> And living people, and the things they understand."

I realize I will never fully understand how much
you suffered alone, but I do know that
I shall never forget thee,
My dear beloved, Dava Lee.

chapter one

When and Why I Chose to Write

It was early November 2008 when the doctor informed Dava and me on Tuesday, the weekly chemo day, that there was a blood clot in the vessels leading to the liver. She was instructed to take blood thinning shots to eliminate the blood clot. The following Saturday, after enjoying an evening with my brother Rob visiting us and spending the night, Dava suddenly became nauseous and threw up a spittle of blood. I immediately called Dr. Van Amburg who was on weekend emergency calls. After being informed of what had just taken place, he said, "Oh shit, go to the emergency room to be checked out and do not take any more blood thinners."

After the emergency room visit and a few more days of not taking any more blood thinners and nearing the noon hour, Dava again became suddenly nauseous, only this time she filled the whole bottom of the bucket with blood and clots of blood. I knew she was very frightened because I, too, was frightened. It was off to the hospital as fast as we could go, and Dava was never to return.

Since I lost my wife in December 2008, I have read a number of books and other writings about loss. When considering the loss of a spouse, a dwelling place is the only choice of words that comes to my mind. When two people are united, and one departs, leaving behind the other half of what was before, the heart still dwells there.

There are these certain events in each one's life that stand out compared to other days, weeks, or even years such as the day one celebrates a sweet sixteenth or telling twenty-first birthday or the day one meets the love of his life. The only day that may be more memorable and reverenced is the day that that precious love is lost. This book results from my continuing search for those exact feelings that will address my loss, and by my expression of these feelings, may connect my soul with persons who trace a similar path.

I have been faced with the closest tangible connection to Dava which were her personal journals penned during her illness. On the inside cover of her first journal, Dava wrote, "This journal is dedicated to anyone who cares to read it." Her entries reveal so much of Dava along with all the trials and tribulations one fighting a terminal illness can experience about life and pending death.

"Of course," it struck me, "her story should be shared!" There are thousands in the same situation who may be unable or unwilling to lay bare their vulnerabilities, the unrelenting loneliness held within, and the struggle to face the reactions to events and people around them. I, too, thought her story was worth telling to help the many who might be timely touched by her testimony: to take each day given until there is simply no more to give.

chapter two

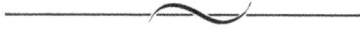

The Beginning of Our Life Together

At this point in the narrative, I think it is necessary to go back to the beginning of our relationship and how I eventually found and managed to marry one of the most beautiful ladies God ever created. Dava was voted the most beautiful girl at De Soto High School in the Class of 1966 Yearbook with a special page featuring her near the back of the book. I went to a Catholic high school, and our yearbook designated no such section as this, and she never once mentioned anything about being pictured in her yearbook in such a fashion. It was only after we were married, and I was paging through her class book that I discovered it. I don't ever remember her even acknowledging this honor, although to me it didn't matter; for I knew she was the most beautiful girl in the school; but to see it listed was certainly amazing. So the next thought should be: how on earth did I manage to date her, let alone marry her? To be truthful, I still haven't figured it out for myself, but I won her heart because I loved her from day one, and we somehow became as one. It was always Gary and Dava after that.

She even waited for me to finish college. Of course, I knew the necessity of having access to a car; but with ten siblings and a few older ones who had their own vehicles, it was difficult to count on my turn to ask to borrow for more than one night every couple of weeks. Not that she would have required that, for she only lived ten blocks from where I lived, but I wanted my own car to take her on dates.

Our first real date to the big city stands out to me because I just got my first car ever midweek, and I asked if she would like to see *The Sound of Music* playing at the St. Louis Theater in St. Louis, and she said yes. Of course, I didn't know anything about cars or too much about the car purchase I had made. The car was owned by a well-known and respected family in De Soto, and it seemed to me to be a good deal, especially since it was a 1957 Chevy. It was a four-door yellow with a white top, dual exhausts, and black and white seats.

On the trip to the city, this beautiful girl of sixteen with thick, long, curly, and reddish- brown hair, those sparkling, almond shaped green eyes, and dressed in a one-piece, shapely dress of pink mohair was sitting right next to me. As we headed up the highway, I began to smell exhaust fumes. Soon Dava began coughing. Out the back window, it looked just like a jet plane streaking down the road, two exhaust pipes pumping out the smoke. Dava assured me that she was fine, but I couldn't help but wonder if maybe I made too quick a deal. In spite of the smoky conditions, we made it to the movie, enjoyed a fabulous dinner, and made it back home. I did eventually correct the exhaust problem with the money I saved on the purchase, but later I could not help but reflect on Dava's thoughtfulness that evening in tolerating such discomfort with such grace.

So now I was off to a good start, completing my college studies and graduating in June 1968. Within that first week home, Dava and I discussed our wedding plans and setting a date of Friday, August 2nd to be married. Later in that month of June, I mentioned to Dava that the Jefferson County Draft Board had contacted me on my status. I was told by the lady at their office that if I wasn't joining a branch of the armed services or joining the National Guard that I would be receiving my draft notice within three to four months. Well, I nearly messed everything up on this particular night by saying that maybe we should reconsider staying with our marriage plans. Dava was hurt so deeply when I, knowing that Vietnam was possibly in the forecast, mentioned the thought that maybe we shouldn't marry until I finished my Army obligation. She just told me to take her home. She had tears in her eyes, but she was very firm in her request. For the eight minutes of drive time hardly a word was spoken, and those came from me. I sincerely thought it was something I needed to address, but I then realized just how much those words about postponing our wedding date had hurt her; so I took her home as she requested.

Luckily for me, my mother was still up when I returned to the house a little earlier than usual. When I told her what had taken place and what I had said to Dava, there was a noticeable, shocked look in her eyes. She said, "Honey, Dava is one of the loveliest persons I have ever met. Are you sure you want it to be like this?" I immediately answered her that I felt so bad, but I really didn't know what was best for us. Then I told her how much I loved Dava, and she could see the sadness in my eyes. I looked at Mom and expressed my thanks to her for listening. I did know what I wanted and what I had to do.

Within thirty minutes having passed since having dropped Dava off at her house, I returned and knocked at the door. Her mother came to the door and asked what was wrong and said that Dava would not come out of her room. I asked if I could talk to her, simply telling her that it was my fault for whatever she was feeling. I tapped on her door and literally begged her to talk with me. She didn't answer until I pleaded with her in apologizing words and with a heartfelt wish to be with her. It was the longest five minutes I had ever lived through, but then she opened her bedroom door. Her face looked so beautiful to me, even with her mascara rolling down her cheeks. We hugged like we had never hugged before, and in one breath, I asked her to forgive me for hurting her so and stated that I couldn't bear to even think of living without her, no matter the circumstances we had to face. As we squeezed one another and both of us shedding tears, we kissed a heavenly kiss; I told her I loved her more than myself. I felt so happy and was so glad I was brought to the real essence of what her love meant to me; from that moment, I have never regretted going back that night. She was, is, and will always be the "One Love" of my life. Dava did forgive me although she occasionally, during our forty years of marriage, brought up the story of that night, maybe just to remind me that I once wavered on her. She would use it at times as a slight nudge to my ego when I thought I was on top of the situation.

Now you need to know a few more things about Dava. She not only had a beautiful outward appearance, but she was also very smart, shy in a sweet way, and very talented in so many ways. For the most part, she had great patience along with persistence, unless I did something totally stupid; even then, she could muster enough stamina to correct my erring ways with respect and kindness.

I'm thinking back to our first Christmas with the first of our daughters, Stephanie, ready to receive toys. We celebrated on Christmas Eve, a tradition my family had practiced since I was a youngster. It was forever to be the best day of the year for our little family. After sharing presents, usually some clothing, books, and if I was on my game, some jewelry for Dava, our attention turned toward getting the toys put together to await Stephanie's visit from Santa. I always sang at Midnight Mass, and Dava stayed home with Stephanie and began assembling the toys. So when I returned around one in the morning, she would save a couple of items for us to assemble together. She soon discovered that the putting together routine was not my forte; for with the first screw put to the wagon handle, I managed to strip and then let the screwdriver slip and scratch my hand. In all honesty, it was only a scratch, but one might have thought I lost a finger. Dava simply suggested I relax and take a break while she went on to complete the assembly. So for her next birthday, I bought her a tool box because if anything in the house needed tender care, she could fix it. Like most of my brothers, I just never acquired that mechanical knowledge for fixing things. I like to think that endeared her to me. I knew that I definitely needed her more than she ever realized.

Dava was the oldest of six children, as opposed to my being the ninth out of eleven. So what's that got to do with the price of tea in China? I don't know; but just maybe she watched her father as he fixed everything; and there is a good possibility that she also inherited many of his talents. She was so adept at doing almost anything with her hands. She could sew as well as anyone. In fact, I can remember her drawing up a design that only a qualified engineer could understand. She made her wedding dress and the bridesmaids' dresses, and everyone thought they were professionally done. She was so proficient in shorthand that if I wanted the words to a song on the radio, she could copy it down as it was playing. A high school friend of hers later told me that Dava was the fastest at shorthand in the class. Her penmanship was elegant, and she was a speedster at typing or drawing almost anything. It was simply remarkable to watch her. And she was always making something. Even while viewing a program on television, she would be knitting a hat for a little one or whatever creation she was thinking about at the time to make for someone as a gift.

Let me continue on thoughts of Dava's creative talents a bit longer with another illustration. I love to share just how talented she was at making or designing almost anything. We moved to Paducah, Kentucky, in 1979 in her thirtieth year. After I became more acquainted with Danny and Lee, our new neighbors, I introduced them to Dava. After some time had passed, and Lee became aware of Dava's varied abilities, Lee asked if Dava would help make some life-sized baby dolls and maybe show and sell them at the largest craft fair around Paducah, held at Kentucky Lake. Well, our four girls were eleven, eight, five, and two at the time, so Dava was a little reluctant to commit herself to such a time-consuming task. But I encouraged her to take part in this creative venture because I knew she enjoyed anything to do with sewing, and creating dolls was right down her alley. It is my recollection that both Dava and Lee agreed to try to make ten each. So I didn't pay a lot of attention to their project for a couple of months, but soon the Saturday arrived for the big craft fair at Kentucky Lake. I wasn't that interested in the fair itself; but when they returned, I was certainly concerned with how things went with the dolls. Well, Dava's dolls sold at one hundred dollars each in like the first two hours, and Lee sold six of hers. Lee remembered how lifelike the expressions on Dava's dolls were and how exacting every feature stood out and exemplified her creative talent.

One week later after Dava had told me the doll making was too demanding of her time, I realized the hundred dollars per doll was actually too low a price. She then informed Lee that though it was a fun project, she just could not continue making them. So on the following Saturday while Dava was grocery shopping and I was at the house with the kids, the phone rang. It was a woman calling from New York City. She asked if she could speak with Dava who always attached a name tag to each doll, naming them and including the words, "Made with Love by Dava." I let her know Dava was out shopping, but then she said that she called to ask Dava to make her two dolls because a friend of hers visiting Kentucky Lake had shown her the dolls she had bought from Dava. After I related my wife's intentions of no longer making the dolls because the time required to finish them was just too demanding, the woman assured me that she would wait as long as necessary, and Dava could charge whatever amount she felt was needed. Then the caller added that she just fell in love with her friend's dolls and relayed how much it would mean to her to have two for her children. I suggested she give me her number, but she said it was long distance, and she would be happy to call back. About an hour later, the lady called from New York, and Dava spoke with her. After the phone conversation, Dava told me that the lady was so nice and complimentary about the dolls she had seen that she told her she would make two for her. I remember Dava's thoughtfulness when she asked the lady if she had any particular names in mind for the dolls. Dava said she was very nice and gave the names she wanted.

In a few days, a check arrived for a hundred twenty-five dollars for each doll, although Dava had told her she would make them for a hundred each, plus she added enough for the shipping and postage to send them. As Dava sat there reading the lady's kind note of appreciation, I just looked at her and was overcome with the thought that she actually touched the heart of a person in New York City and was gracious enough to understand that the lady really appreciated everything that went into making those dolls. And my now grownup children reminded me just a few years ago that they still have possession of two dolls their mother made for them. One's name is Bartholomew Aloysius. I guess maybe it was named for the boy we never had, and the Aloysius part just happens to be my middle name; the other was named Pearl, a very pretty, little black doll and one of the favorites.

chapter three

My Family Meets Dava

It wasn't a wholly one-sided mismatch that I may appear to have set up here. Since childhood, I had worked hard, having lost my father to leukemia at the tender age of six. My family also consisted of eight brothers and two sisters and the most caring and loving mom anyone could have wanted in that situation. Believe me when I say that our family turned out to be well respected in our small-town community of De Soto, Missouri.

All of us grew up and knew how to earn a living by working hard and by always lending a hand with household chores. But more importantly, we learned how to love one another in special bond of family. There was never a dull moment in the Doyen household. We knew how to have fun amongst ourselves or with anyone who visited our home. Early on, I'm sure, many of us were a bit naive and uncertain about what the future held for us, but the desire to achieve all we were capable of came almost as automatic as flipping a light switch. We all inherited good body fitness and a genuine concern for each other and for others.

Soon after that glorious, fumed-filled trip to the St. Louis Theater in St. Louis, I thought it was time for me to introduce Dava to my mother. You need to know that Mom lost the one, true love of her life, Ralph, when he was only forty-two years old; and she was left with eleven children, with Judy the youngest just nine months old. Mom knew she had to be strong of mind and heart and not give up. So even though the oldest siblings were old enough to help out, Mom realized that this huge responsibility rested largely on her shoulders, and she never shrank from it. And now I could hardly wait to show her the pretty, sweet girl I had sought and found.

It was just after Dava's family had finished their dinner that I arrived to pick her up for our date to attend a dancing party in town. I'm quite certain we did not tell her father about going dancing. He was a very strict Baptist, and I wasn't sure he would approve at that point in time. When Dava scooted over next to me in the car, I mentioned that I wanted her to meet my mom before we headed south for the dance party. She said she would love to meet her. So it was off to my house. When we entered the front door, there were sounds of laughter, talking, and more laughter as seven of my brothers and two sisters were eating dinner.

Dava must have thought she had just entered an army canteen with all the commotion. Dava was dressed to kill as the saying goes, and before I could introduce her to Mom who was standing near the stove, all my brothers were checking out my beautiful and fabulous date and asking to be introduced. Of course, they were polite and gentlemanly in every way.

Mom caught my eye, and I said, "I wanted to introduce Dava Copeland to you first," and she walked over to us. Mom made anyone in her presence welcomed with her gentle smile, and Dava, I think at that very moment knew she was seeing a family that would love her just as I did. One of my brothers got me to the side to ask me where I found someone as beautiful as Dava, and I replied, "Right here in De Soto." She did look like an Italian beauty. Many thought she was identical in looks to Sophia Loren, and she was.

If all the stars were not aligned by this time to know that we belonged together, I soon discovered that Dava and I had had a brief meeting when we were both babies. One night while I was waiting on Dava to get ready to go out, I spent some time chatting with her mother. Before I could tell her about my family, she interrupted me and said, "I knew your dad and mom many years ago when we were first married. Your dad rented to David and me a room in your house for a couple of months when Dava's dad returned from the Navy." So I found out that Dava and I had actually shared a playpen sixteen years ago when we lived in a big two story house at the north end of De Soto. The stars and planets must have all been aligned for this reunion to have happened.

chapter four

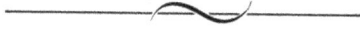

Joined Together in Marriage

It wasn't long after, that the wedding date we had set for August 2, 1968, arrived. Dava chose her sister Jeanne as her maid of honor and my youngest sister Judy as a bridesmaid. At the same time, I picked Charlie, my next oldest brother, as my best man and my next older brother, Pat, as the groomsman.

Dava used the small apartment of my great Aunt Emmie, who was considered by my family a living saint, to get dressed for the wedding. It made Aunt Emmie so delighted that she was in the midst of such a wonderful occasion, that the bride to be was at her little place across from the Catholic Church. One would have had to know Aunt Emmie to understand how precious the atmosphere was for her. She was of a diminutive stature but certainly not in her presence and state of being. She had been serving her whole life working in a seminary kitchen, feeding the young men studying for the priesthood. Many of the priests still remembered her as being diligent, gentle, and kind. Emmie had very little formal education but always spoke in a reverent and kind way, and these attributes are what Dava most appreciated in her, as we all did. Aunt Emmie may have attended other weddings, I don't know, but this time she had the bride to be at her home, and she loved it all. Some may have thought her somewhat old-fashioned, but Dava loved her for her simplicity and was so pleased to have Emmie with her charming little ways present while she dressed for her wedding night. It meant more to me than she ever knew although I had nothing to do with setting this up. Mom or my older sister, Mary Lee, must have suggested it. But I was told from childhood to respect Aunt Emmie because my dad had told all in the family that she was a very special and beautiful person.

After the ceremony, it was off to the reception where we gathered with family and friends for a few hours before heading out for our honeymoon. Well, I hadn't planned for an exotic place to spend our honeymoon. I figured the excitement of our first night together would be terrific wherever we ended up, but we were headed to Springfield, Missouri, where I spent my last two years finishing college. It's a three-hour drive to get there, and it was around ten o'clock before we left the family gathering. I suggested we stop at the nearest hotel along Route 66, so you see I can get pretty romantic when the situation calls for it.

Driving down Route 66, we arrived in Cuba, Missouri, and spotted a huge, really nice-looking hotel at that exit. It was now nearing the eleventh hour, and I was the only person at the reception desk asking for a room. The attendant said he was completely filled up; no room left at the inn. I was still dressed in my tuxedo and told him it was my wedding night. He looked at me with a drooping jaw and began telling me if I had been here ten minutes earlier, he could have given me the suite, but he had just given it to an older couple because it was all he had left to offer. So then I asked if there was another hotel close by. He said it would be in Rolla, another fifty-minute drive, but there was a motel about two hundred yards away. He admitted that it wasn't much, but at least I could probably get a room there.

After thanking him for the help, Dava and I went to the motel to check it out. The attendant was right. It wasn't much to look at, but the lady attendant was very nice, and sure enough, she had a room available. We took it. It was like going from the Royal Astoria to a Motel Six within two hundred yards. If only I had planned better, we could have had a very nice suite; but as small as the place was, it had the necessary furniture, and it made for a memorable night forever.

chapter five

~

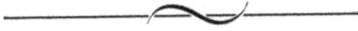

Our New Life Together Interrupted

The first five months Dava and I lived in a small apartment in Hillsboro, a small town not far from De Soto, our first dwelling place together as man and wife. She thrived on making each day special for us. On occasion, she would surprise me with a candlelit dinner, and then I knew for sure it was going to be a thrilling night. And she did it all so naturally. She was born to be the best homemaker, and that's why her being the mother of our children was the one thing I most respected and appreciated in her.

In December 1968, she had one of those candlelit dinners, only this time she had something extra special to share with me. She told me that she was pregnant. I certainly had no idea, but I remember how her face glowed while delivering this wonderful news. We were both obviously excited and extremely happy. Even the reality of my being drafted, with a January 8th Army obligation staring at us, couldn't ruin this night together.

So January came, and I was off to Fort Leonard Wood in southwest Missouri for basic training. Dava and I had discussed where she would live while I was serving our country. She would stay with my mom and the remaining siblings still living at the house. It was the perfect place to be, for Mom loved having her around, and Dava enjoyed being spoiled a bit by so many. And for me, I felt that she was happy and secure, and that meant everything to me.

I had no time between basic and infantry training at Fort Ord in California, so my sisters brought Dava and Mom to the St. Louis airport. We now had at least a couple of hours together before my departure. Then in May 1969, I received a two week leave before heading to Vietnam. Dava was now five months pregnant, but we made the most of those two weeks. In fact, there was a photo snapped by either Mom or Judy of Dava coming into my arms with both of us smiling; all of our four daughters have told me that it is their very favorite. Maybe it's because I was so happy to have her there in my arms, and it shows. Now it has become my favorite too.

For any soldier away from home, nothing, I mean nothing, comes close to mail call. I just heard in the past month from a dear friend of mine that he was given a free trip with others to Washington, D.C. from the Veterans Honor Flight. The highlight of the whole experience was when the people in charge yelled out, "mail call," and gave him his huge bundle of letters. The one reason I bring this up was Dava's diligence in writing to me during my tour in Vietnam. She wrote nearly every day, many pages; if I didn't receive one on a particular day, I would get two or three the next. Believe me, not everybody was so lucky. I knew exactly how many backup letters were coming by just counting the days since the last one which I read over and over. My mom wrote at least once a week also, but to know I was assured of getting a letter almost every day sustained me and gave me every desire to want to make it back home. I'm quite sure that Dava did not realize the importance and the value her daily writing provided in sustaining me throughout these very arduous and often perilous times. After a few weeks in Vietnam, I wrote and told her that her letters were as important as breathing is to my lungs. Again, in contrast, I saw many soldiers who might receive a letter every two weeks. Dava was my lifeline even over there.

There is one more important story to tell of Dava during my Army days. After returning from Vietnam with six months of duty remaining, we had thirty days of leave time before we left to report to Fort Rucker, Alabama. We were very fortunate to spend this month away from the military in an apartment after our future sister-in-law, Vi, informed us that it was available for this short period of time. When

I arrived from Vietnam, she had made this apartment into a home. Well, I guess if she could manage to travel to Hawaii in January with our four-month-old Stephanie to spend a week with me, she could do almost anything she set her mind to do.

After settling in at Fort Rucker in housing off base, Dava and I had a memorable experience. It was Thanksgiving week of 1970, and after moving off base, I became close friends with many fellow Vietnam returnees, but there was one in particular. Amos Ferrantio came with his family as a first generation of Americans from Portugal, and he was just nineteen years old while I was twenty-four. His family lived far off in Massachusetts, and here he was like us stationed about as far south as one can get. So I asked Dava about inviting him to our house for Thanksgiving dinner instead of his having to eat in the Army mess hall. She of course agreed, and we all enjoyed one of Dava's expertly prepared meals and a lot of great conversation. Amos spent nearly the whole day with us before I took him back to the base. At the time, it never occurred to me what this day with Dava and me really meant to Amos. It was in late 2004, Dava called me at work from our house in Raintree subdivision west of Hillsboro to say she had received a call from Amos Ferrantio in Boston. She gave me the number he left with her, and I soon returned his call, just very anxious to connect with a dear friend of thirty-five years ago.

After thanking me so graciously for being a mentor to him at that youthful age back in 1970, he progressed to the main reason for his call which was that Thanksgiving Day. He said that visit to our place on Thanksgiving Day was one day he would never forget. He then added that Dava fixed the most delicious Thanksgiving meal he has ever had even to this day. He continued to thank me and Dava again and again and said that we made him feel like he was a member of the family, and he would always remember Dava and me for as long as he lived.

All of what Amos remembered happened in a one bedroom, concrete, block house; yet he recalled most of all the smell from Dava's cooking and the entire atmosphere of love and togetherness that made it one of the best days in his life. From our phone conversation, I recall his saying that as he looked back on that day, he realized what we had together as a family. That was the driving force for him to want the same. I get a tingling in my spine when I recall that phone conversation. I befriended him, but Dava made it a memorable moment in his life forever.

chapter six

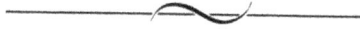

Early Signs Something Was Wrong

That word forever brings me back to where I left off when possibly the first signs of an illness was apparent to Dava, but surely everything seemed fine to me. We had built the house of our dreams in 1999 at Raintree Plantation, at a lake resort near Hillsboro, Missouri. Dava had always wanted a huge front porch with enough room for plenty of seating space to view the beauties of nature and just feel the gentle breezes of the spring, and this house filled all those requirements perfectly.

It was the summer of 2006. Dava, our four now fully-grown daughters, and I had seven wonderful Christmas celebrations there by then. The view from the front porch encompassed the one-hundred-and-thirty-acre lake. All our neighbors were especially friendly people. Then just after dinner on a hot July evening, Dava said, "Let's sell the house and move back to De Soto," which was only ten miles from Raintree. I tried to convince her that we had a beautiful home, that our daughters often visited, and that this was the house we have always wanted. She answered so succinctly, almost as if she had been rehearsing this conversation in her mind for quite a while. She then replied, "If something were to happen to you, I wouldn't want to live here, and if something were to happen to me, you probably wouldn't want to live here." She went on to say that she could have everything packed during the day and have the house ready to put up for sale within a couple of days. When I suggested waiting till next spring, that it might be a better time, she answered, "I really would like to list it right away." So we spent a good part of the evening and into the night figuring numbers and eventually concluded that we would call an agent in the morning.

Dava did time the market right, and we were able to nearly get our asking price within two months. If we had waited till spring when the housing market was slowing down, we would have received less. Some very dear ladies who were sisters and also close friends of the family let us use their house during the winter months while they were in Florida.

Within about three months in early January 2007, we found a newly built house nearing completion at Lake Summer Set in De Soto. The builder was in the driveway about ready to call it a day when I suggested we stop to check out the interior; the exterior looked great. Dava protested a little at first, realizing it was the first house we had seen that was for sale, but I convinced her that the builder would show us the house before he listed it. On entering the house with the builder within hearing distance, Dava said, "I love it." I'm sure that was music to his ears. I cringed a little at that point, and after a walk through, I informed the owner that we would think about it. Within three weeks, we were moving into our last house. It was January 28, 2007.

There was another instance which only came to make sense to me much later, when Dava told me early one morning as I was leaving for work, "It feels like something inside me is eating at my insides." I recall turning back to her and asking what she had said. I heard what was said but did not know what she meant because she said it so casually and then added, " Oh, never mind, it's just me."

This last occasion was sometime in June 2007, and by early August, I began noticing that Dava seemed worn out on some days. She loved watching two of our grand-daughters each day for the past few years while their mothers worked during the school year. Since the new school year was fast approaching, I shared with my daughters the fact that their mom appeared very tired these days and that I did not think she should take on this responsibility. As it turned out, the school decided to go to full days for the preschoolers instead of their attending half days, so everything worked out to ease the strain on Dava. She had had knee surgery in May of that year, so I continued to suspect that most of the weariness was due to that.

The next indication that something was not right with Dava also came in August. She asked me if I thought her eyes had a yellow look to them. I stared deeply into those gorgeous eyes, but I truly could not see any yellowing. My daughters shared with me that their mother had also asked them if they saw any yellow in her eyes. Like me, they had not noticed any change in their mom's eyes, Dava somehow knew that her eyes did have some difference about them. So now when I look back to this time, I believe she honestly knew something in her system was not right, but not enough to sound an alarm.

Fall had arrived, and it was Sunday, the third weekend in September. After returning from eleven o'clock Mass, we settled in the living room. The football games were on television, but I had my eyes in the Sunday newspaper. Dava was crocheting.

It wasn't too long before she said, "Honey, I have this pain on my left side beneath my rib cage." After asking how long she had the pain and proceeding to ask her if she wanted me to take her to the emergency room to check things out, she just said, "No, it's been there for a while." She further explained that maybe the pain began when she moved the nightstand a couple of weeks ago. So we talked about it for a bit, and then she assured me everything was fine.

There was never a better moment for me to remember than Dava and I talking and laughing when just the two of us were in a room. We would discuss everything from the kids, to literature, to things that occurred throughout the week. What made it extra special was when something I said made her laugh, and it had to be funny. She did not laugh just to please. It had to really hit the funny bone. No one could ever see a more beautiful smile than Dava could produce, with her glowing emerald eyes thrown in for an encore.

Around two o'clock the following Wednesday afternoon, the phone rang at Mueller Electric, the furniture and appliance business I took over from my sister Mary Lee. It was Dava telling me she had become terribly sick at her stomach. She described how she had thrown up, and that it was like a projectile just spewing out. Her voice had a real sense of being scared by the experience, and she mentioned her intention of calling her doctor to see if she could get in to see him tomorrow, and she asked if I could go with her. I told her that she should call him, and we would go up together, and that I would be home right away.

When I reached the house, Dava looked as good as always but described how suddenly the nausea came upon her and how forceful the moment was for her. I could see the concern on her face and hear the timorous edge to her voice.

Something else I noticed was the box of Prilosec lying on the table next to her chair. I asked her when she started using that medicine. She informed me that she had indigestion, and one of our daughters gave her the remainder of her package to see if it would relieve the acid reflux. So, again we thought maybe this was the problem she was dealing with, and maybe today's episode was actually due to an acid reflux problem.

So on Thursday, September 27th, I drove Dava to see her doctor, Dr. Phillips, at St Luke's Hospital and Medical Buildings in St. Louis. After the visit, Dava told me that she had related in detail what had happened on Wednesday, about the throwing up incident and the severe acid reflux she had been experiencing, but I learned later that she had not mentioned anything about the pain under her rib cage. Since we were both scheduled for our annual physicals the next week, the doctor prescribed some medicine for the acid reflux and told her he would see how she was doing next week. We left the doctor's office, stopped by for a late lunch, and headed home feeling things were back to normal, or at least I did.

Dava was not one to complain too much. She used to say that my colds always seemed more severe than the ones she had, and I thought they were as well. So with her new prescribed medicine and a good week with no new incidents of being sick, we were quite certain the acid reflux was the cause. Everything seemed fine.

chapter seven

---~---

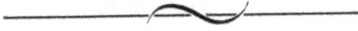

Coming to Grips with the "C" Word

On Thursday, October 4th, Dava and I again headed to St. Luke's Medical Center for our semi-annual checkups. That infamous October 4th day will forever be emblazoned in my brain, as we sat together in the waiting room to see our doctors. Dava was called first to see Dr. Phillips as I waited to be called by Dr. Ellison. Within about five to ten minutes, Dava came from her physical accompanied by her nurse, and the nurse informed me that when I was finished with my doctor's visit to come over to the emergency room. The doctor had ordered some tests to be performed on Dava. I asked if I should just go with her now, but the nurse said that the tests would take a while and to just come over after I was finished with my doctor visit.

Well, I was in and out within about ten minutes, and everything went well with my visit. As fast as I could, I hurried over to the adjoining hospital, down the hallways following the signs that led me to the emergency room. When I arrived there, Dava was sitting up in her bed in a small emergency room cubicle, and I asked her why Dr. Phillips wanted to run the tests. She told me that after she had informed him about the pain in her lower chest area that he wanted to make sure there wasn't a blood clot in her lungs.

The hospital laboratory had already completed an ultrasound when I arrived. I asked Dava how she felt since I still did not have any idea anything was seriously wrong and because she appeared in good spirits and did not look sick. But then a male nurse came to her bedside and said that Dr Phillips ordered a CT scan with fluids. I wasn't really thinking very well when I asked the nurse how long might the scanning procedure take; for we hadn't eaten since early morning, and it was now around three in the afternoon. He answered, "Well, I'm sorry, but she needs the scan right now." I assured him that I understood, not realizing the magnitude of the moment.

Soon after, another nurse came with fluids for Dava to ingest before the scan could be taken. It was a thick, milky substance that probably tasted horrible, and she had a whole bottle of it to swallow. Dava suggested I go get something to eat because it was going to take thirty to sixty minutes to down all the fluids, and that I could be back before the scan started. It seems more than a bit thoughtless to me now that I agreed to go grab a bite to eat. I went to my car and called our daughter Andrea, the third oldest, who was at the store and told her that her mother had to undergo some tests, so it might take a while before we would get back to De Soto.

So I left the hospital and drove about three miles to find a restaurant. I ate quickly and was headed back in thirty minutes. But the drive back to the hospital at that time of day made it seem like I was never going to get back in time for the scan. The cars were moving more like a bunch of turtles. I finally got parked at the hospital and ran as fast as I could run to get to Dava. The first thing I asked her was if she had the scan, and she told me she had not, but that Dr. Phillips had just left. I couldn't believe I had left and missed the doctor. Then she informed me that Dr. Phillips said he had ordered the CT scan because the ultrasound showed that something was up with the pancreas. I then expressed my disappointment in myself for not being there with her before the doctor left.

Then my cell phone rang. It was our youngest daughter, Sarah, calling about her mom and asking me if we knew anything. I began telling her that she was given an ultrasound, and the doctor said that something was up with the pancreas. Sarah immediately asked me if anyone had mentioned the "C" word. I answered no and confirmed only what I had told her earlier. The nurse's aide came to take

Dava for her CT scan, and I told Sarah the minute we had any news, I would let all our girls know what was going on.

It didn't seem like it took all that long for the CT scan procedure to be completed. The aides were rolling Dava back to the emergency room cubicle, and I was holding her hand as we traveled down the hallway corridors. It was around five-thirty that early evening, and the original doctor's appointment had been at one o'clock. As Dava lay in the bed, I was asking her how she felt, and all she said was that the fluids she had to drink were horrible. At this point, I kept thinking that soon this will be over, and we can go home to spend a normal and quiet evening together.

It was now approaching the eight o'clock hour, and when we were not talking, I was pacing the small area of the room staring at the doctors, nurses, and other staff, looking at their screens; I was wondering if they had totally forgotten about us. Suddenly I saw one of the doctors rise up, but instead of coming in our direction, he was heading toward the lab or screening room. Dava, I knew, had to be hungry although I don't recall her saying anything about it. I kept wondering what was taking so long. We had been here most of the day. Just before eight o'clock, the emergency room doctor showed up at our cubicle. He stood to the right of Dava's bed as she greeted him. I was on the other side of the bed. The doctor began saying he was sorry it had taken so long, but the lab has been extra busy today.

He also informed us that he wanted to check with the lab again before he came to us with the results and that he realized we had been waiting a very long time. Then he looked directly at Dava and said, "Anything inside the pancreas is supposed to be only of a liquid nature, and you have a solid mass, and I'm sorry." As he turned to walk away, he said, "You can call your doctor in the morning; he will have all the pictures of the scan and the written results."

One would have to have been there to see the pain in this doctor's eyes when he uttered the words "I'm sorry" to us; for no sooner than he spoke those words, I looked at Dava to see a single tear drop from her eye and roll gently down her face. The doctor more than likely has had to deliver news like this to many others. I think that he turned after saying that to gather himself, as I no doubt would have done because the tear affected me as I'm sure it affected him. I can't remember what we said to one another after the doctor left, just that we hugged one another and Dava said, "Let's go home."

At this point, there were a thousand thoughts running through my mind when Dava very calmly said, "We need to stop at the desk to pay our copay." Grace and beauty together were sitting in that wheelchair. So after I brought the car to the door, the nurse flipped up the foot stands on the wheelchair as I opened the car door to begin the mysterious ride home. Why was it mysterious? It was mysterious because neither of us could recall much of what was said to each other on the hour-long drive from St. Luke's. I do know there were tears shed; but at that moment in time, what does anyone know what to say; for hope is all we had left to consider. We certainly didn't want the lever of hope to get any lower in our spirits than it already was. The thought that the solid mass was possibly not malignant was running through my mind.

Soon after leaving the hospital, Dava called and informed our four daughters as to what had been presented to us. To this very day, this one-hour drive home is a blur except for the phone calls to the kids. My mind seemed to be darting in all directions, mainly trying to digest what may lie ahead of us, that neither of us could begin or dare to think about after this very long and arduous day. The news we received that evening didn't sound promising at all, but we for sure did not want to face our future without a positive thought or two. We had been through nine long hours, but the day ended up centered around these words, "You have a solid mass inside your pancreas, and I'm sorry."

It was nine o'clock before we finally arrived home. Dava went toward the bathroom, and I made a call to my sister, Mary Lee, to tell her of our situation. She said that our daughter Andrea had called and told her the news. After asking if there was anything she could do, I answered by saying that we just needed time to comprehend everything that was said and done today. Soon Dava was back in our living room, and we just gathered on the sofa, held each other, talking some, and tearing up some. The doctor had not mentioned the "C" word, and neither did we, hoping against hope that there was still a chance, slim as it might be, that the tumor in the pancreas was not malignant.

So we went to bed just so we could lie together with our arms wrapped around each other. Maybe it was a blessing that the day had worn on us so much, that sleep was what we needed, but it was difficult to come by. It was at least an hour, maybe more, before I drifted off into sleep. As we were holding each other, all that was going through my mind was that the yesterdays seemed to have disappeared. It was what happened today, October 4, 2007, that flashed in my brain, over and over again, actually over my whole body.

chapter eight

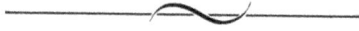

Treatments to Lift the Lever of Hope

Early Friday morning, Dava received a phone call from Dr. Phillips informing her that there was indeed a tumor in her pancreas. After she asked him a few questions, he said that he was setting her up with an oncologist for the following Wednesday and also gave her the name of a renowned pancreatic surgeon should that be a future possibility. Neither of us had any appetite. Only the food for thought was our diet at this point. We needed some answers to our deep concerns developing over the difficult news we had to digest from yesterday. Dava and I now knew that she would be facing a tough uphill battle. We were truly devastated with this latest news. Is it a case of being sick, very sick, or terminally sick? These were the questions facing us.

So after the call from Dr. Phillips, I suggested to Dava that we try to get in before Wednesday. When I called to ask for an earlier appointment, the receptionist advised me to call first thing on Monday, the 8th of October. I told her I would call first thing on Monday. I was able to move the date of our first visit to the oncologist one day earlier to Tuesday with the head of the department, Dr. Van Amburg. It may not seem like much of a difference, but we were literally in a state of the unknown and scared to discuss too much before we had more knowledge of our situation from our doctor.

On Saturday, we drove to a shopping mall in south St. Louis County, I guessed as a distraction; but Dava had a purpose in mind. She wanted to purchase a journal. As soon as we entered the Border's Bookstore, she headed straight for the journal section and bought the first of her journal books. I wasn't thinking anything about such a companion book, but I wasn't the one diagnosed with a tumor in my pancreas. From that day onward, there were her daily journal entries, the exception being when she was too sick to write. As I watched her writing in her journal, I told her that whatever she wrote would be to herself as she wrote. I wanted her every thought and feeling to be exposed without having to share anything with me. By now I have read and reread many times all three and a half journals she filled up with her many daily routines but also some very poignant statements concerning life and death. As I later read through the journals, I placed asterisks on certain passages that sometimes encouraged laughter and others that brought forth tears; for only Dava could convey truly and in depth her suffering and loneliness. As terrible as the physical pain was at times, the pain of the mental torment may have been the greater tragedy of this disease.

One would need to understand that Dava's family was attached to every fiber of her being. And if one was so fortunate as to be a part in that fiber, what a lucky person one was. Dava mentioned in one section of a journal entry that all she wanted was to be a wife, a mother, and grandmother; then after a few sentences, that being a great grandmother would still be a wish she hoped to see. She excelled in all these categories with the exception of becoming a great grandmother. She never had the chance to become a great grandmother. So when that fateful day came, where it was known that a terminal cancer would take her, everyone connected to her fiber of being was heartbroken and began a sort of wondering in a desert existence.

Oh, we had not given up hope that there was the possibility that the mass was a non-malignant tumor, but that wasn't in question after our first oncologist meeting with Dr. Van Amburg. He was a tall, stately man, probably around sixty years of age with a vast amount of experience in his specialty. He also had a very personable doctor-to-patient demeanor about him. He first stated that he definitely believed the tumor to be cancerous because of its jagged appearance, and then came a worse blow to our ears when he noted that there was a spot on the liver which was most probably inoperable. He then asked Dava if she wanted to view the results of the scan on his computer. She replied, "I always like to look at pictures." He even printed the pictures for us, so we could see everything he was pointing to. As for me, I was just contemplating what procedures the doctor would suggest to take on this battle. Dr. Van Amburg wanted an MRI of the liver spot and a PET scan of the pancreas and liver areas to evaluate the significance of the spreading cancer. So now we knew that we were dealing with pancreatic cancer that had spread to the liver. The hope lever just dropped lower in reality, but not in our willingness to fight the good fight as Dylan Thomas begged in "Do Not Go Gently into That Good Night."

My brother John and sister Mary Lee were with us on the first visit and were there throughout the course of Dava's treatment. In fact, many of my family attended Dava's office visits. Sometimes three or four were there, but always two or more. Soon the nurses started saying, "Dava and her entourage." Terry, the doctor's receptionist, commented to me how faithfully Dava's family was there to support her. I respectfully corrected him by saying that this was my family, and they were there for us to the very end of our journey. My sister, Mary Lee, treated us to a very good lunch after each weekly session. But the news from that first visit was tough to fathom. We were holding out some hope, but now it appeared that only a miracle or an undiscovered cure would be where any hope might be found.

Going back almost a year and a half, I remembered an incident in 2006 that suddenly came to mind. This gentleman was a customer of mine, and I hadn't seen him for nearly a year. In May of that year, he was in my furniture store, and immediately I went toward him. He looked very thin. When I greeted him and asked what had happened, he informed me that he had been dealing with pancreatic cancer the past few months, but he was hopeful that he was in remission. He passed away thirty days later. That was just fifteen months before Dava's diagnosis. I couldn't forget the toll this cancer took on his body. His spirits that day were surprisingly still good, but he didn't win the battle with this cancer. As we soon discovered, not many do.

Just now I was checking Dava's first journal entry to make sure the dates used were correct, and on her October 11, 2007, entry, she had a clipping from *Parade Magazine* listing the death of Luciano Pavarotti, who died of pancreatic cancer at the age of seventy-one on September 6, 2007. Yes, pancreatic cancer or any cancer consumes one's existence, especially for one in the throes of the disease and also for those loved ones surrounding that person. When the diagnosis is terminal, everything gets magnified. It's like having a lot of rainy days and just waiting for a ray of sunshine now and then.

Dava and I had again made the trip to St. Luke's Hospital on Wednesday, October 10th for Dava to receive the PET scan, which to the best of my knowledge, radiates a picture of the cancer's hot spots. They show up in illuminated, bright red colors. The pancreas tumor for certain was brightly lit up, due to its four centimeters plus size, about the size of a walnut. The liver having a thirteen-millimeter size was much less, but the doctor wanted an MRI on the liver spot and a biopsy of the pancreas tumor. Terry, the receptionist, said he would schedule an appointment for Monday, but I informed him that Dr. Van Amburg wanted the tests as soon as possible. We were conferring with Terry from home on Friday morning, and he graciously said he would get it today if we could be there before noon. I told him we would leave right away and thanked him for working it out. I was thinking that one day lost in treatment might mean a lot, and the sooner the doctor had the exact scope of the matter, the sooner he could begin his treatment of Dava.

Considering the first visit on September 27th was followed by the infamous October 4th diagnosis, then the October 9th PET scan, and last but not least the October 12th MRI and biopsy, to say we were in a state of frenzy would probably sound redundant. The MRI went quickly, but the biopsy was very hard on Dava. Thank God she had a wonderful male nurse named David Lopez though his nickname he said was Davo. Dava and Davo hit it off instantly with their nearly shared names. He was obviously Hispanic, and Dava went into quite a description of him in her journal of just how nice and macho of a man he was. Davo called me in to be with Dava as they were preparing to put a twenty-gauge needle just under the rib cage, reaching all the way down to her back where the pancreas lies. I was glad Davo was there for her: for later she commented to me and in her journal that no matter the circumstances, she would not have this procedure again. It was simply the most excruciating for her.

Again, my brother Denis, his wife Gail, and my brother Rob, who drove from Columbia, Missouri, were with us on this very difficult day. At the time, I wondered if enough appreciation was shown to those who were always there when Dava and I needed them. I am here to say now, I don't know how one gets through times like these without such loving family support. I just need to read in Dava's writings to realize just how much this family support meant to her.

It was the following Monday night when we received visits from Ralph and Betty, Denny and Gail, John and Onie, all of them my older brothers and their wives, plus all of our children came out along with the grandkids. A number of floral bouquets expressing get well messages and lots of thoughts and prayers had arrived that day. The younger grandchildren had not yet been told of the severity of their grandmother's condition or that she had been diagnosed with pancreatic cancer. Our granddaughters, Kelsey and Elizabeth, were thirteen at the time, and both truly loved being around their grandmother. Dava suggested to our daughters to at least wait until the Hannah Montana concert coming up on October 18th, was over to tell them. But who receives flowers and bouquets on a day when there is nothing to celebrate?

Just a week before on Saturday, the parish at St. Rose of Lima church in De Soto held a healing service Mass in the morning for anyone who was ill or suffering. Dava and I attended. It was the first time many of our friends were able to show their support for Dava on a personal one-to-one visit. Monsignor Buchheit, a close friend of our family, presided over the service, and afterward he came over to Dava and me saying, "Dying is not the worst thing." The words definitely were forcing reality, but Dava laughed and actually noted in her journal that, "Actually in some instances maybe dying is the best thing." It sort of lightened up the atmosphere for Dava even though we weren't anywhere near accepting that end.

chapter nine

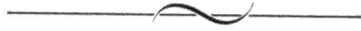

Trying Times Amidst
Diminishing Hopes

Returning back to that Monday before the visits from family that evening, Dava and I were expecting a call from Dr. Van Amburg giving us the results of the PET scan, MRI, and biopsy. After receiving a call from my sister Mary Lee that she had a pot of potato soup for us, I told Dava and her mom and dad, who were visiting from Fredericktown forty miles south, that I would get our prescriptions picked up and bring the potato soup back for lunch.

It was nearing the one o'clock hour when I arrived at my sister's to get the soup when her phone rang. It was Dava. She began telling me that the doctor had called and said the spot on the liver was cancerous, an adenocarcinoma from the pancreas. It was another devastating surreal moment. I told Mary Lee that I needed to go to Dava right away and left without anything except the urge to be by her side. I knew she needed me then, and for certain I needed her. Dava's journal entry conveys the overall feelings much better than I can:

> Mom held me, and Dad wept ever so silently into his red bandanna handkerchief. I called Mary Lee's to see if Gary had made it to her house, and Gary answered the phone. I told him what the doctor said. He told me he would be right home. When he got here, Mom was holding me, then Gary knelt and put his arms around me while I just let it all out.

It was oneness of being. I didn't have the disease, but I would have rather accepted the cancer on myself than to see my love suffer so.

I have just paused from my writing for fifteen minutes and picked up a companion of mine to read, *Leaves of Grass* by Walt Whitman. I have turned to him many times the past eight years, but this section suddenly opened itself to me. Whitman had attended a church service where the minister's topic was "The Rounded Catalogue Divine Complete," but as Whitman listened, the minister in his sermon, according to Whitman, included in letter and spirit only the aesthetic description of life's experiences and entirely ignored what Whitman states in the following excerpt:

"The devilish and the dark, the dying and diseased, the crazed, prisoners in jail, the horrible, rank, malignant, venom and filth, serpents, the ravenous sharks, liars, the dissolute; the barren soil, the evil men, the slag and hideous rot . . ."

Though I shortened the verse somewhat, Whitman placed *malignant* right where it should be, in the middle. The cancer, the evil one, destroys its victims and affects the loved ones surrounding him or her in a very debilitating and tragic way.

One night as we were sleeping, Dava sat up in bed with her arms wrapped around her knees. I awoke and asked if there was anything wrong, and she told me that this was the only position that would help relieve some of the pain in her lower back. Without thinking first, I mentioned how she had been doing this off and on since August. I then asked her if the pain was the reason then because I thought she was sitting up due to her acid reflux. Dava then admitted that the pain in her lower back was the reason for her sitting up in bed even back then. The big difference now was that the pain would probably get worse, not better. I went to the kitchen to grab two Tylenol tablets which helped her rest a little easier. My thoughts were running wild, for I had not realized in those earlier months the pain she was bearing.

Dava asked me to walk with her into the living room, and we continued to walk in the dark. It was about one in the morning. We walked for maybe fifteen minutes through the hallway, around the living room, the kitchen and dining room over and over. She was in front with me behind with hands around her waist, guided by the ray of nightlights. We were talking and wondering how all of this came upon us. Dava then became angry with the cancer and uttered "I'm so mad. I feel I could run my fist through the wall." We continued our walking a while longer and then sat together on the sofa in the dark with only the nightlights staring at us. After several minutes, she said, "Maybe a cup of hot, green tea would be good," and I agreed that would be just the perfect thing to do. So I made us two cups, and we settled in each other's arms for nearly an hour before she was able to go back to bed. That was a night I will always remember so vividly, and from then on Dava's determination seldom faltered. Oh, there were plenty of setbacks, and she was well aware of what lay ahead, but a night that started so heavily filled with emotions seemed to end with the desire to share the love we had now in this moment.

At first look, Dr. Van Amburg was in hopes of using surgical radiation to eliminate the tumor on the liver, but after consultation with the surgeon and radiologist, he decided it would be too dangerous to attempt. The tumor was located near the top of the liver, and the fear of burning through the diaphragm or lung would be catastrophic. Again the hope lever descended for us, but Dava confided to me that she was relieved that she would not have to undergo the procedure. During this visit, we met the nurse practitioner, Debbie, who told us that the doctor's staff was setting up Dava's treatment schedule, beginning with chemotherapy. The specific type of chemo used for pancreatic cancer is designated as *Gemzar*, a name we had never heard before, and suddenly it became a word used time and again in our household conversations. When Dava asked when the first treatment would begin, Debbie replied, "Today."

Going from the doctor's office door, Dava and I entered this spacious, sunlit room with huge comfortable chairs of fifteen to twenty in number, and all the patients were hooked up to what is called a chemo drip bag. Four to five nurses were on duty to check on each cancer patient. Soon one of the nurses introduced herself to us and began informing us how the procedure would be done. First, Dava was given steroid pills to help counteract the ensuing nausea, followed by the infamous needle into the vein in order to release, drip by drip, the noxious but vigorous cancer fighter.

My brother John and I sat in front of Dava and began chatting about almost anything that came to mind while Dava seemed to wonder in silent thought about just what this chemical emptying into her vein and body would do for her; for Dava seldom, if ever, permitted any substance known to be harmful to her health to enter. She enjoyed eating fruits of all kinds, like apples, grapes, and peaches which were her favorite. Nearly every fresh fruit available was almost a daily habit with her, and now this substance flowing through her body was poisonous and yet vital. Some patients were given two drip bottles which for some was a three-week supply, but Dava had one and within an hour all of its contents went from the bottle into her system. The fact that others around her were doing what she was having to do may have eased the anguish that living with chemo would bear on her state of being. After the needle was removed, she was finished with her first chemo treatment only to return every Tuesday for the remainder of her life.

Thus far I have not mentioned our daughters in much detail only because I know how devastated they were. It was difficult and sad to see how they came to accept the thought of their mom having pancreatic cancer. Stephanie, the oldest, was thirty-eight at this time. She was born while I was serving in an infantry company in Vietnam. Carrie's birth was my first experience in the delivery room where I tried to help Dava ease the pain of childbirth. They both did quite well without much help from me. Andrea's birth was induced on the due date, and everything happened during normal, daylight hours, as opposed to Carrie who was born after midnight. Then Dava's doctor suggested that maybe, due to her varicose veins, she should consider tubal ligation which she proceeded to do. But after eighteen months, our daughter Sarah came into this world. Were we surprised? Yes, but what a wonderful and blessed surprise she turned out to be. All four of our girls and their mom had such a special bond of mother and daughter love for one another. I especially remember the holiday season when Dava would leave with the girls for a day of Christmas shopping which they all enjoyed, and they would all come home dragging, except for their mom, after eight hours. Oh, for one more holiday season just to experience that.

Needless to say, our daughters could not do enough for their mother during her illness, and they knew that I was always there for her, so just maybe that made the journey a little less painful for them. They often fixed our dinners for us and were at the house almost daily to visit with their mom and bringing the grandkids along which made Dava happy. Fortunately for me, I can see Dava in all of them, in their features and a lot in their mannerisms. How lucky we were to have our daughters; for sometimes it would seem as Dava shared with them that she was not sick at all. I would sit back and just watch them and see her spirits rise and wonder how things looked so right in my sight, and yet I knew the pain inside was so severe as it had been just a few hours ago.

As I am writing at this moment in time, the door to my deck is open; and I'm viewing the backyard with the beautiful redbuds staring at me. They're almost the same color that the American Cancer Society uses to signify pancreatic cancer. They'll soon be followed by the flowering dogwoods which are wild and grow in large numbers along the border of the yard. Other than the Christmas season, the springtime was Dava's favorite as well as mine, although I think autumn is definitely its equal. Actually, Dava's illness caused her to really appreciate all the daylight hours, for the nighttime seemed a lonely time for her, especially when I fell asleep lying next to her. She felt alone in her spirit. Again her journal entry explains the feelings better:

> *Then off to bed for another span of darkness when I feel so alone for some reason. Gary will be right next to me, but when I know he is asleep, I just feel scared and every thought in the world crosses my mind – until I might drift off for an hour or so, each time waking, hoping the daylight hour is near.*

Earlier that same day, Dava was online and had viewed cases of pancreatic cancer patients from the Mayo Clinic site. She noted that most of the patients with stage IV pancreatic cancer had barely survived six months. That alone would be enough to make a saint a little fearful; in fact, I had read at the time that Cardinal Bernardin of Chicago, after having pancreatic surgery six months prior, when notified that it had returned, was devastated. So I think Dava was handling herself bravely indeed.

There were nights when I would awake to find Dava spending the midnight hours sitting in the recliner I had brought home for her to spend any waking hours close to me in our bedroom. Only once did I ask her what she was thinking about because she answered, "If you don't know, then I can't explain it." Of course, I knew some of what I expected would be going on in the mind of a person facing a stage IV cancer diagnosis, but I'm not sure I understood the surrounding loneliness that came upon her in the dark. She noted in her journal on a night when all our girls and grandkids prepared a dinner and stayed with us for a few hours just wanting to be with her that, "At times when all the family gathered together supping and talking, I felt like a little dot on the wall, not wanting to participate, or probably wishing more that I could be happier, after all, everyone was here just for me."

Now more than ever I'm more capable of understanding the essence of inner loneliness that thrives deep into one's state of being. For each year that lapses, another stripe is earned in my realization of how life is without my love to share it. In October 2014, I wrote down my thoughts on how alone one can be which I titled, "Alone, Thoughts of Dava:"

"What word might compare? Would it be: forlorn, weary, forgotten, absent, to just name a few? Does it always associate itself with sadness? No, but there is an association. The impact of being alone surely seems greater when alone follows

a true bonding of love; then separation exists. I might conjecture that the supreme state of being alone is in our thoughts of death; for in death no one can fully understand its impact, except the sufferer. All that is outside this realm is cast aside for those in death's throes; for the mind of the sufferer must absorb a life's completion coming to an end. What thoughts must cross in exhausting flourishes of feeling, as Dava once acknowledged, as a dot on the wall to all others about you. Alone even in a gathering of those loved ones, it seems so ironic, but it happens this way. Philosophy, religion, a belief system, do they quell this darkened room or add to the confusion?"

My love's death haunts my spirit at times to the point of being alone in crowds, feeling forlorn. It's as though a sword is piercing my heart when I touch something of hers, see something she wrote, or imagine her lying on her side of the bed.

For months after entering the house after darkness fell, for it was early December when I lost her, I walked to our bedroom to put my lips to hers, only to touch a soft pillow instead, to leave only a tear there. Alone, the tear soon dried, waiting for the next one the following night. Absence, it's more than absence because there is the thought of nevermore, nevermore, absolutely nevermore."

Once when I was reading *The Selected Letters of John Keats,* my favorite poet, I shared with Dava a line he wrote to Fanny Brawne, the love of his life, "A person in health as you are can have no conception of the horrors that nerves and a temper like mine go through."

Later I read in Dava's journal entry, written in late November 2007, where she states, *"Gary is reading to me from his Keats book – you will see the quote at the top of the page – how true and how exact those words written by a person who was the one dealing with an incurable illness. Keats hit the nail on the head with that statement."*

chapter ten

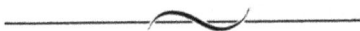

Dava's First Extended Hospital Stay

Our first extended hospital stay began with the one in November 2007. Dava was in so much pain one night, I could scarcely console her. Trying to move at all made her agonize in complete misery. We had no clue what brought this on, but she was suffering, and the pain would not let up. I called the doctor's night line, and he suggested we go to the emergency room or wait till morning to see Dr. Van Amburg. It was already after midnight hours, so Dava got as comfortable as she could on the sofa, and that's how we passed the night. Since she did not have a fever, we decided to wait till morning.

The first thing in the morning, I called the doctor's office and was told to come up right away. When we arrived, the doctor's staff immediately got a wheelchair for Dava because she appeared so frail. We rolled right through the waiting room into the doctor's office, and Debbie, the nurse practitioner, met us there. Dava had some difficulty moving onto the examining table; after just minutes, Debbie said that the problem was either a blood clot or pneumonia; so off to the emergency room we went to find out.

The doctor who came to her bed side in the emergency room was the same doctor who had given us the results on the night of October 4th. He was first to make the connection to us saying, "I'm the one who was with you that night. I'll take good care of you." It was very comforting to see him go into action. He told us in just a few minutes that it was pneumonia and that he would start administering the antibiotics immediately. I guessed that the first three chemo treatments had weakened her resistance.

We stayed on the seventh floor, the cancer floor at St. Luke's, for four days in a single room because being on chemo meant she could not be exposed to anyone who was also ill. I stayed with her around the clock and slept on a cot the staff provided for me. Some may think it was admirable of me to be there for her, but really, it was the only place I wanted to be. And I was just thankful I had this time to give to her when she needed me. There were many in the same situation, but they had to make time after going to work or caring for children, so I was the fortunate one. I was able to stay with the one person I wanted to be with day and night.

Here are a few remembrances of the hospital stay that

come to mind. First, there was the priest serving as the chaplain at St Luke's and his humble demeanor that made his presence all the more welcoming. When he entered Dava's room for the first time, she was sleeping, and I greeted him while preparing to wake her, for I thought she would like to meet him. He simply said to me, "Just let her rest for now. It's an honor to just be in her presence." That certainly made for an immediate connection between us, and he was absolutely correct with those words, for I too felt the same in her presence once he had spoken. Later we got to know him, and he said that he was here for us if we should ever need him. No doubt he was appointed to this job of hospital chaplain because he knew how to relate to patients dealing with cancer. Each time Dava had to enter the hospital, he came by to see her, and his genuine kindness and humility were always present.

Another memorable moment, thanks to Dava's journal entry, was my helping her bathe the following morning. Here's how she related it:

"Took a shower and Gary helped me wash – he said I looked "sexy" ooh! I sure don't feel "sexy." Finally I had a bowel movement Hoorah! Felt better than sex."

Through all the sickness and pain, she still never lost her humanness or her sense of living despite the ravages of the cancer that dwelt within her.

Later that day, our niece Erica and her daughter Ryann came to visit Dava. That was after visits from our daughters Andrea and Stephanie who brought her crossword puzzle books which she loved to work. Andrea also painted her toenails. At the end of the day, Dava wrote all this down in her journal and added this precious closing:

"Keep thinking about Ryann patting my bed--- she would just stop whatever she was doing about every five minutes and come over and pat my covers."

Ryann was three years old at the time.

chapter eleven

Remembering the Love and Support for Dava

After being released from the hospital on Monday, Dava proceeded to have a good week, and on Thursday, she and I went to a St. Louis County mall with my sister Mary Lee. They both liked the Bath & Body Works store, and while shopping, an elderly, little lady mentioned to Dava that she liked the fragrance she had chosen. Dava's journal entry reads:

"A little lady said she thought the fragrance we had chosen was her favorite too. I said it must be our age is why we preferred it over the others. She said I didn't look that old and that she was 92. She looked 80 to me. We got to talking & somehow got on my health – she asked me my name and said her son's name is David. She also said she would remember me in her prayers – she was the sweetest person. I somehow feel we were meant to meet, my guardian angel, maybe."

The following few nights Dava wrote in her journal some thought-provoking lines that express very well how challenging it is for one suffering as she did. On November 10, 2007, she writes:

I've been feeling sorry for myself the last few days – so selfish of me. Every little ache or pain I think the worst. I worry about what's going to happen after I'm gone. Like how silly is that – after all, I won't be here to know. I worry about Gary, and who might take my place – if they will love and care for him the way he deserves. If anything does happen, I want him to find someone special to love again – Oh, no I don't! I worry about each of the girls, knowing how alike and how different their emotions will be – I worry about the grand-children, their futures. Not meaning to show favoritism, but I especially worry about Abby – we all do. I worry about my parents, don't want to cause them any worry. I just seem to worry about everyone and everything – Time to take my chemo pill, Goodnight.

Then three nights later she writes:

"Oh Dear God, just give me the strength to get thru this, but I mostly pray for my faith to be strengthened. Gary is reading "Romeo and Juliet" – he said it was our story – he's so great."

Then one night we attended a fundraiser, a wine tasting event, our daughter Andrea had planned to benefit the school. We went for about an hour, but I guess that was more than enough, for she wrote:

"I felt and I don't know why, like I was a circus item on display. Everyone was just being nice but they were only coming up to me and saying their prayers were with me. I appreciate their love and concern, I guess I just don't like being the center of attention. And Gary seemed to enjoy himself tasting the wine and talking with others. I guess I wanted to have fun & just couldn't. All the other women looked so healthy & pretty & I just didn't even want them to say hello to us. I knew they meant well & I'm not unappreciative but I just feel so much as being on exhibition – well, it's as though others know I've got something a lot worse than I myself realize. I was cold and all wrapped up in a dark cape – no wonder people were coming up to me---I must have appeared as though I had one leg in the grave – I'm sorry."

We had sat at a table with family, and many did come up to Dava to wish her well and let her know that their thoughts and prayers would be with her. And I probably acted my normal self, talking with the guests who came by our table and enjoying the wine without realizing that Dava was feeling like that dot on the wall. Though she was with mostly family and friends and could enjoy the moment, her moments were being consumed and never to return.

After going to bed that evening around eleven o'clock,

Dava began talking in her sleep, at times shouting out and tossing in the bed. I awoke and just gently stroked her cheek telling her she was having a dream. Her journal entry reads:

"In the middle of the night I felt something crawling on my face – finally realized it was Gary's hand moving back and forth across my cheek – he said I had had a dream and was saying "Dad." I remember having a dream and saying that in the dream but I can't remember what the dream was about or why I was shouting Dad."

Sometime in late October 2007, Dava called two of the doctors she had been seeing. One was Dr. Morley, her gynecologist, and the other was Dr. Tull who operated on her knee in May of that year before any of the cancer news was known. Her journal entry relates her conversations with the doctors:

"I told them I guess my reason for calling other than looking for another shoulder to lean on, was with Dr. Morley about having already canceled two appointments because of my knee, and I felt I needed to cancel my appt. on Oct. 30th. With Dr. Tull I just wanted to make my appt. with him easier, so I wouldn't fall apart on my visit with him next month on the 29th. I told him hopefully my hair will not have fallen out yet, he laughed. I thanked them both for listening to my personal trials and tribulations and wished them both a Happy

Thanksgiving. Dr. Morley said her thoughts and prayers were with me and that I should do nothing but concentrate on resting and getting better. Dr. Tull said he would keep me in his prayers & said if there was anything at all that they could do to just let them know – that he sure hated to hear the news and that we would talk about it more when I come in on the 29th. I told him I hadn't even thought about my knee, and again he laughed."

Well about a week before the Nov. 29th appointment with Dr Tull, Dava called his office, and she writes:

"I called Dr. Tull's office, at first the receptionist said he was in surgery today, booked up tomorrow and with the holiday week, I probably wouldn't be able to see him this week. Then quickly she said, Just a moment, when she came back to the phone said she had spoken with Kate who told her to have me call or the nurse in chemo call as soon as I was finished with chemo to see if I will feel like going over to see Dr. Tull, which Jan said she realized would probably be afternoon right after my scheduled chemo treatment. She said she would keep my file on her desk and that Dr. Tull would be made aware of my phone call. At first Jan seemed rough spoken but she turned out to be one of the nicest persons."

That tells me that Dr. Tull had informed his nurse Kate that if Dava needed to see him to make any accommodations necessary. Both Dava and I thought this to be a very kind gesture on his part, and when we did arrive at his office, he took her right away and was interested in just how well she was doing. He and his office personnel were really terrific in seeing after her needs at this difficult period, and I especially thank Dr. Tull for his thoughtfulness and kindness.

I feel it is worth sharing a few more journal entries before I continue the progress of our journey. Dava had told Dr. Van Amburg that the needle pricks in the vein were getting to be too much for her and asked if she was a candidate for a port to inject the chemo fluids. He definitely agreed and set up the procedure to get it done as soon as possible. So on November 20th she was scheduled for the surgery and writes:

"There I talked with the surgeon Dr. Gronin, probably in his 30's. He was the surgeon who had looked over my original CT scan results with Dr. Van Amburg. I asked him if there was any hope. He said it was in a bad area, my pancreas tumor, because if it had been in the head of the pancreas it would have given early warning signs such as jaundice or yellowing of the whites of the eyes. Also in the body where my tumor is located, there were no signs until the tumor reached a size that finally caused pressure on nearby areas causing my back to hurt. I told him I was never in really great pain, which he said was another sign that does not show itself for a while. He

concluded by saying he had seen patients given prolonged lives w/chemo treatments and some better quality of life."

Dava shared his views later that evening with me, and I'm sure he was giving her the facts as they were, and having the tumor in the body of the pancreas allowed it to grow unnoticed to where its size caused it to rub against the multitude of nerves near the spinal cord, and even worse, gave it time to spread to the liver. That is exactly what makes it so deadly, the stealthy nature of the disease.

During Dava's port surgery, a number of my family were there, including my brother, Rob, who drove in from Columbia, Missouri. When Rob's daughter, Danielle, just began working, Rob had given her his car and bought a used car for himself at the time. The reason I mention that part about the car is to make it easier to understand Dava's journal entry of that day:

"Rob came from Columbia to be with us on this day, making the trip with his not so new car. He is staying the night – he is so pleasant to be with –he rode up with us at 7:20 AM and stayed throughout the entire ordeal. He could have easily gone home with John, or I'm sure Mary Lee would have driven up to get him, but he is just a good genuine, wanting to be there kind of guy. I feel so at ease when he is around."

Another person I need to recognize as being especially

supportive and consoling for Dava is the son of my brother John, Fr. Mitch Doyen, who was ordained a Catholic priest in 1991. My mother, who had always wished and prayed for one of the family to enter the religious life, would have been very proud of him. It was just a few weeks after the cancer diagnosis that Mitch called and visited Dava and me and offered to have a Mass for Dava. He was so gentle in his person and spoke so eloquently as he dedicated the Mass and blessed her with the Sacrament of the Healing. This service touched Dava deeply as it did all of us present. All the children, grandchildren, some of their friends, and many of my brothers and sisters were there that Saturday night. I was not as diligent as Dava at recording events in my journal, but I did write about that night with Fr. Mitch and family saying:

> "The celebration of the Mass meant so much to us all, but most importantly for whom it was intended, Dava. There was a tinge of sadness throughout and I especially noticed the tears in our youngest daughter, Sarah's eyes, and my sister Judy was gently wiping a tear from her eye as Fr. Mitch dedicated the Mass, his chosen Scriptures, and during the Sacrament of Healing. Dava later told me she enjoyed having everyone here for this occasion and how she now dreads the beginning of the night, but that night she slept like a baby."

Sometime in early 2007, a fellow infantryman whom I

served with in Vietnam came into the furniture store with his wife. It had been thirty-seven years since we last saw one another. In fact, we didn't recognize each other until I handed him by business card. He then asked me if I knew who he was. I suggested he give me a hint. As soon as he mentioned Vietnam, I said, "Larry Keating." So after that day, we visited each other on numerous occasions during that year, and in October, I told him the tragic news of Dava's illness. It was sometime in November that he gave me the name and phone number of a person referred to him by another one of our Vietnam acquaintances. This person had stage IV cancer and was given little hope of surviving, yet he was still alive because he had switched courses and adopted an Indian regimen that he said completely reduced the size of his tumors dramatically.

After relating to Dava what Larry had told me, I suggested that I call, so we could hear firsthand what this guy experienced. He was living in Florida and was aware that I might be calling. He was very forthright in saying he had taken treatments for months, and eventually the oncologist informed him that the chemo wasn't working any longer, and the tumors were growing larger. He then gave me the title of a book, *The Cure for All Cancers*, that had formulas to gather and consume. He concluded by saying it has so far worked for him. This was November, and the doctors had told him in April that he probably had a couple of months to live. Dava was sitting in the living room as we talked on the phone, and I asked him if he would share his story with her. He assured us that he wasn't trying to convince anyone to go this route but would try to help in any way, that it was a last resort for him and so far it had worked. So Dava did talk with him for a few minutes and thanked him for sharing his story and wished him well. I also thanked him for his time and asked if I could call again if I had any more questions about his routine. After I mentioned getting all the required mixtures gathered may be difficult, he told me he would help out in any way he could, but again he stated he wasn't wanting to convey that it was something the medical profession approved of, but that it was his one alternative to the bad news he was given in April. Dava's journal entry on the subject reads as follows:

> *"Gary's Army buddy called w/news that another friend had taken an herbal drink which made tumors on his liver completely disappear. I checked online about the herbal remedy Gary's friend's friend suggested. I don't think (I mean I know) I will not be doing this regimen. One ingredient, wormwood caused hallucinations, seizures, psychosis, and death. We are still going to check out an organic food store tomorrow for some other possibilities."*

I did talk to that friend of a friend one last time a week or so later and ordered the book. I never followed up on anything pertaining to the Indian remedy, but at times I sometimes catch myself wondering if it might have worked; then again, if it had caused even worse, adverse effects, I would never have forgiven myself. Dava was quite clear she was not going there at all. I did ask about him in 2009, and he was still alive and living in Canada. So I lost track of him, but hopefully he is still carrying on. I must admit he was direct with us and only said it was working for him, so God bless him for his willingness to help.

chapter twelve

~

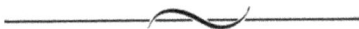

Our Last Christmas Season with Dava

Now the holidays were approaching with Thanksgiving coming on fast while Christmas was in view, too. Dava's youngest brother, Scott, wanted to visit her, and he offered to prepare the Thanksgiving meal and all that went with it, of course with the help from his wife, Carol. Dava was very happy to be able to share this holiday with her brother, his wife, and their two children, Sydney and Samantha. Scott really did perform all the preparations for the Thanksgiving meal to a tee. He was up at six o'clock preparing the turkey with Dava alongside taking it all in. I can't be sure of all the activity that morning because they didn't wake me. It was about eight-thirty before I awoke to join them.

Everything appeared to have gone very well that day. Dava summarized in her journal:

"Our Thanksgiving dinner turned out great. Scott's turkey

was so moist, and Carol's cheese French bread and cranberry sauce were delicious, and our girls, Andrea cooked the dressing to perfection, Steph's mashed potatoes and Sarah's green bean casserole were almost all eaten, and Carrie's sweet potatoes and pumpkin pies were raved about, and she had decorated the house beautifully for Christmas – We looked at pictures of my side of the family, that was really fun – I guess because it's Scott's family too. – Everyone is gone now, it's just my honey and me. It was a hectic but beautiful holiday – just pray I'll be here for next year."

The following Tuesday, we again were heading to Dr. Van Amburg's and Dava's entry reads:

"Today is my 6th chemo treatment – then I guess we'll wait & see what the next CT scan shows in a week or so – I'm so afraid – why? – I don't know – maybe I'm afraid of more bad news, but how much worse can it be than what I've already received."

So she finished the second session of three chemo treatments each, and then came the results of the CT scan. From Dava and my perspective, the report wasn't bad, in the sense that the tumors were kept in check. The Gemzar was doing what the doctors hoped it would do. There was another measurement referred to as a *cancer marker*. My basic understanding of the marker was that it gives the number of the new cancer cells being produced. Back in

October the cancer marker was at 468, and now it measured 41. I'm not sure whether Dava or myself actually knew what this all meant in the larger scope of things, but we were in need of some good news to shout to the roof tops, and this was it.

I asked Dava if she felt good enough, that we should go out to celebrate. Even an hour or two of celebration was what we needed, just the two of us. She smiled and said she needed a few minutes to get ready. It didn't take her long, and she looked gorgeous. And her reaction via her journal was, *"Gary thought I looked 'ravishing.' It's amazing what a little lipstick can do."* We proceeded to find a quaint, little restaurant where I proposed a toast to the terrific cancer marker number 41, and we clinked our glasses and followed that with a kiss to the lips. What a little good news could do for our spirits in the midst of so much bad news. It was amazing to have that little bit of good news as a reprieve.

Well, there were not many days to actually make us feel like celebrating, for it was difficult to find moments that would make us jubilant when we could readily see the road was pretty rough up ahead. In fact, a few were just the opposite, sort of a feeling like the glass was half empty. But really, they were few, and now I'm not referring to the bad days when Dava was suffering so or extremely sick but days when she was down in spirit. Dava's journal tells of one particular night that conveys it better:

"Last night before bedtime I really showed myself – I know I made Gary feel like hell – only he can know what we talked about. We didn't say one word from our house to Mary Lee's this morning, and what made it worse was that I was in the backseat! All because I was feeling inadequate and accused him of wanting someone with more energy and free of any 'having to deal with this crazy ordeal' we're going thru."

Truthfully, it was one of those times when Dava needed to get angry with the cancer, and no matter the assurances I gave her that we were in this together, she still needed to get her frustrations of the past two months of fighting the disease out of her system. By the way, there were a few times when she actually preferred riding in the backseat, especially when she had to drink the fluids in preparation for a CT scan, but there were not many, and that was the only time she rode in the backseat to my sister's house. I reveal this above entry from her journal to show how a serious illness can easily make a person feel like a burden on everyone around them although I and all those who loved her never considered Dava a burden. But believe me, the making-up the following night was worth the wait. It was fantastic.

Now at this moment in time I am thinking if I had simply shared Shakespeare's sonnet 116, nothing more would have been needed:

"Let me not to the marriage of true minds
Admit impediments. Love is not love
Which alters when it alteration finds,
Or bends with the remover to remove.
Oh no, it is an ever-fixed mark
That looks on tempests and is never shaken;
It is the star to every wand'ring bark,
Whose worth's unknown, although his height be taken.
Love's not Time's fool, though rosy lips and cheeks
Within his bending sickle's compass come.
Love alters not with his brief hours and weeks,
But bears it out even to the edge of doom.
If this be error and upon me proved,
I never writ, nor no man ever loved."

Somewhere I read or someone shared that being the caregiver can be as difficult on a person as the one with the illness. That is just not the case, for it was out of love that I was able to give Dava the support, not once feeling the pains and pangs of the disease. Dava suffered so many days, and yet her strong will to live for those whom she loved was beyond measure. It's hard for me to list each agonizing event, but there were many. Usually on or about the third day after each week's chemo session, Dava would get very weak, for her whole system was changed by the Gemzar flowing throughout her body. One day as Dava lay on the sofa, she suddenly reversed her position every couple of minutes because she was so miserable. I remember my sister Mary Lee called to ask how Dava was doing, and I simply said that she was totally in misery, and I didn't know how to help her. She came right over to our house, and both of us tried to make things better for Dava, but the pain and sickness she felt would not cease. This went on for maybe an hour or more before Dava was finally worn out and able to rest, still in pain, but the overall sickness let up for a while. Mary Lee was washing her face as I brushed her hair with my hands trying to relieve her misery. Sometimes the effects of the cancer had its way with her; but even though she had a weakened immune system, she would struggle through it until eventually the cancer ceased its fight. I don't know how many times she suffered within herself just reclining on the sofa praying the pain would go away.

Dava said many times that I was too eager to suggest taking her pain medicine, and no doubt I often did sound like a broken record on the subject. She disliked the idea of spending her waking hours in a daze; so many times she just bore the pain without letting on unless it got to the point where it was excruciating. She also had to face the realization that the situation would only progress and get worse with time which had to weigh heavily on her mind. That's my reasoning in saying that the sufferer has the most difficult and challenging task, just trying to survive when all the odds are fighting against all that one wishes for in that condition which is peace of mind and body. That is why she wanted her faith strengthened. She had to find that inner fortitude, for no one, as Keats told Fanny Brawne, can comprehend what the one suffering is having to cope with when the other one is in good health. So she could only ultimately turn to God, sometimes asking and other times thanking Him, whatever the situation called for at any given moment. She showed her love for everyone as best she could throughout these most trying times, and I tried to express my love for her over and over. Beyond all that, she was the epitome of great courage, stamina, and acceptance in carrying on.

Christmas was coming, and Dava was in the midst of her third session of chemotherapy. She always wanted things to be just so and to express her love to anyone entering our home. This December would be different for her because her energy level was operating far below the norm. As I stated earlier, Christmas Eve night was always celebrated with the girls, the grandchildren, my brother Charlie, and Mary Lee. Our daughters took over the décorating of the house. It was indeed festive but was missing Dava's unique touch, but everyone understood.

One particular moment comes to mind during our Christmas Eve family get-together. Everyone had gathered, and all the gifts, as usual, were under the tree. I noticed, and there was a photo snapped of Dava, laying her head against the pillowed sectional with her eyes closed at the height of our exchanging gifts. The chemo's effect had taken its toll, and for a few moments, Dava just drifted off into sleep during all the commotion. As much as she loved this night for all the love it entailed, her body for a brief, few moments needed rest. I can't begin to comprehend what she was having to deal with, for I was acting the role I always did on this night, giving out the gifts to the children. And this was to be our final Christmas together although neither of us thought this was to be the last.

When reminiscing on our Christmas celebrations through the years, there was one feature we as a family always looked forward to and that was viewing the classic film *It's a Wonderful Life* which had become a family routine as Dava and I approached our late thirties. But since 2008, I most often watch it alone. It speaks to me of the happiest and most enjoyable times with Dava, as well as the most difficult and trying times during her battle with pancreatic cancer.

Suddenly, Mary has become the central character for me to watch, how she desires George's attention but is forever, it seems, a young woman whose love at times goes unanswered. There is one scene where George doesn't even consider the notion of ever settling down with her or anyone else. After arguing, Mary asks him why he just doesn't leave; as he goes out the door, she removes a favorite vinyl record that was playing and shatters it against the record player. I can see Dava having the exact same response had I acted as George did because, remember, she almost did when I suggested we postpone our wedding plans as I was awaiting my draft notice.

Then there is George in the bar scene, asking if there is anyone up there to help him when he felt that he was at the end of his rope. No, I wasn't at the end of my rope, nor was it a bar scene, but I was pleading with someone above to intervene, so Dava could live and be with me. Instead of the noisy bar room, it was our lying closely together in our bed; when I knew she was sleeping, I would silently pray and weep, my head resting on her pillow listening to each whispering breath and imagining all sorts of outcomes, and none that were very good.

George is back on the bridge. The snow again begins to fall as he is telling God that he is willing to accept anything to have his family back, no matter the challenges confronting him. George was given a reprieve and was reunited with Mary and the kids. This is where our stories differ. Like George, I had a similar request, but a terminal illness makes it much more difficult to persuade anyone above to come to the rescue. I do believe in miracles, but how the miracle was to be played out was beyond my comprehension. The only way I had of seizing on this desire was just a future life with Dava, of having her to hold and be with me for as long as was possible.

I prayed, hoped, and knew that when I entered the house that lonely night, just a short year later and shouted out, "Dava, kids, where's your mother?" that the only sound I would hear at all was the resounding of my own voice. If I had started to ascend the stairs and grabbed the loose post knob, I would have reacted as George did much earlier in the movie when he threatened to throw it. Indeed, I would have thrown that kindred knob as hard and as far as I could.

And yet with the passage of time, I'm so thankful and feel so blessed that Dava was so much a part of my life that I would do exactly what George did at the end of the movie. I would kiss that beloved, kindred knob. That beautiful character Mary, played by Donna Reed who also succumbed to pancreatic cancer, was indeed George's lifeline throughout, and Dava was mine and remains mine. And now I realize I *did* receive my Christmas miracle, for Dava gave me a wonderful life.

As the year was coming to an end, there were still so many questions left unanswered and scenarios too difficult to imagine that even the thought of counting down time in Times Square seemed ironic for us. So what is this obsession with time all about? I would venture to say that time for most of us is the period when we first realize we *are* until the time we know that soon we will not be, for time is not a universal requirement, especially where eternity enters the conversation. In Ecclesiastes, we read there is "a time to reap and a time to sow, a time to live and a time to die," and those times are all related to earthly, living things.

I remember one afternoon Dava shared that she was really not afraid of dying. It was the heartbreak of leaving all those whom she loved behind. Not being a philosophy major, I found it difficult to respond. So more from the heart than the brain, I attempted to ease her mind. I said to her that I recalled a biblical text that states that in God's realm of eternity, one day is as a thousand years. So whoever of our loved ones should leave us behind that before that day has ended, it would be but a fraction of a second until all would be united. Whether that is the case or not, who really knows? But I was sincere in believing this would be what time in eternity appears to me to be. Dava gently smiled, and we talked of other things.

Between Christmas and New Year's, we were waiting the arrival of my sister, Judy, and her husband, Mark, from California. They wanted to spend most of their time spoiling Dava and me, and just their being here for Dava did that, but in addition to being there, they prepared many meals, and all the delicacies were their forte. It was a big lift to our spirits knowing that they were spending their time, energy, and loving gestures in every way possible to make the holiday season a meaningful time for us, especially for

Dava.

On New Year's Eve, we gathered at our daughter Carrie's house with all our girls' families, Mary Lee, Charlie, Rob, Judy, and Mark to eat, play board games, and bring in the New Year of 2008. While we were playing board games, with Dava on one side and me on the other, I continually looked her way to see how the night was going for her. It was a time for some fun, but questions lingered in my thoughts throughout the evening. With all those who loved her so much surrounding her, was that inner loneliness still present? Was she feeling as a dot on the wall? I knew how these past three months consumed our world, but to a much greater extent, how they must have occupied her every thought.

When we returned to our house with Rob who was spending the night, it was a little after 12:30. We all decided to call it a night and headed to bed. The New Year, 2008, had arrived. As Dava and I sat up facing each other in our bed, we began talking about the toll the past three months had taken on us and trying to contemplate what the year ahead may have in store for us. Dava's journal entry for January 1, 2008:

"Gary and I talked for an hour. It was just so hard being with everyone at Carrie's – I feel it may have been the last New Year's Eve we will all have spent together. Oh Dear Father in Heaven, I need more time with these I love."

Dava had such remarkable strength. With all the fears facing her, her humor surfaced frequently. She noted in her journal about Judy and Mark's visit this way: *"They're spoiling me terribly, and I think I like it!"* And when I was getting dressed to attend weekend Mass—the weather not being the best, she stayed home—and, she thought I took extra care in my preparations before leaving for church. She writes:

> *"Gary really looked "snazzy", he even polished his shoes – I accused him of not looking so nice when we go together. Someday soon he'll finally be able to dress the way he wants to without any nagging! The women will be flocking to his handsome charm, though he doesn't match colors too well by himself."*

When I first read this entry after her passing, it was with a mixture of her sense of humor coming through but also a mighty dose of reality. In actuality, I really should not have bothered to polish my shoes, not that they didn't need it; but concerning myself with such a trivial exercise was a bit self-centered of me as her world was falling in on her.

We began the new year with fears and doubts but also with the firm conviction that our love for one another and the support of family and friends would see us through the coming year despite all of its trials. We were now anxiously awaiting the arrival in the second week of January of my brother, Jim, and his wife, Sandra, from California. Dava was already a quarter of the way through her second journal and holding her own with the cancer. The treatments were taking their toll, but her appearance and outward spirits seemed remarkable for all that she had confronted in the past three and a half months. At times inwardly she must have felt an awareness that others were thinking only of the worse possible outcomes for her since pancreatic cancer usually produces such results. As Dava reflected in her journal around this period of time:

> "I don't seem to enter as enthusiastically as I did in the first journal – I seem mad or just mean in this one – maybe it's the stages of my condition making me feel so differently. People may ask or think, why don't you just get over it and let us get on with our lives – Well, I can't get over it! I'm sorry if I'm putting on a false front, but that's what it takes to get thru this."

This statement takes me back to Cardinal Bernardin's assistant who stated that the Cardinal was devastated to know that his pancreatic cancer had returned and was terminal. Dava would have been the last person to put on a false front. She confronted her debilitating condition with strength and a strong resolve to live her life for those whom she loved or anyone who came into contact with her as she had always done. Few could know the difficult days it took to process all she had running through her mind. I once suggested to her, after her sharing her thoughts with me, that this was her "Agony in the Garden." As I understand it, He knew what the verdict would be in the end, and yet those around Him were able to sleep. It makes me so sad to think of all those times that I was able to sleep as she sat quietly alone grasping the fullness of the rain clouds hovering above her and still was able to function and deliver that beautiful and glowing smile for so many.

On January 8th, Jim and Sandra arrived in St. Louis and met us at St. Luke's just as we were finishing a chemo treatment session. We went for a lunch, and they came with us to our house to spend the night. It brought back to mind the feelings we had during the holidays, having them share their time with us and providing comfort, plus a whole lot of spoiling. Dava's entry that evening reads:

"Sandra is so sweet – she comes right in – started cleaning and waiting on me. She was tired from their 5:00 AM flight from LA, but you sure wouldn't know it. Jim stayed up with me, being very patient with me and my computer – how pleasant that they're here."

Besides doing a lot of chores, including laundry, vacuuming, making up the beds, just having them to visit and give us their support was their greatest gift. Oh, and they outdid themselves on dinners for us. On the day they left,

Jim brought dinner out for us. When Jim dropped off the food, he hugged Dava, expressing his love and support as he said goodbye. The scene brings tears to my eyes to this day.

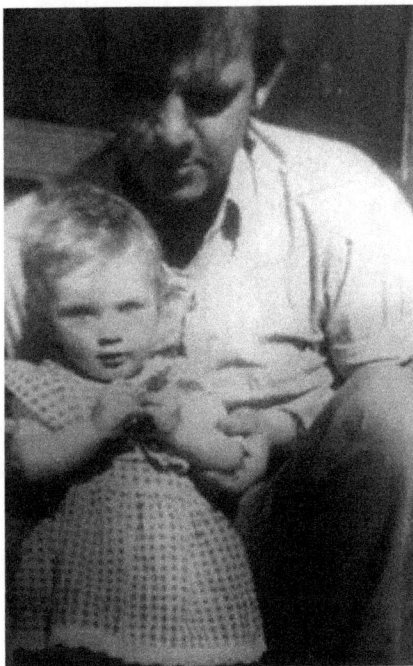

Dava with her father.

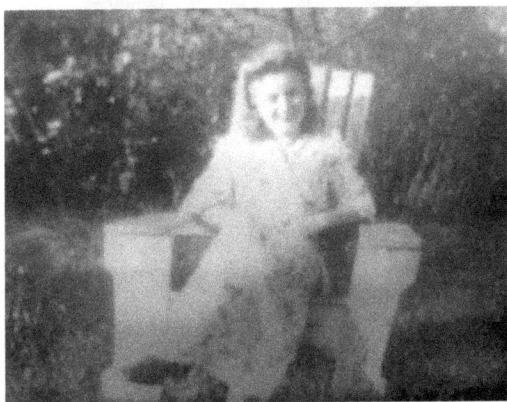

Dava's mother.

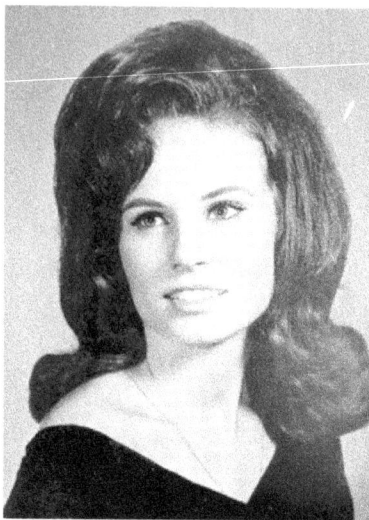

Dava Copeland voted "Most Beautiful." DeSoto High School. (1966)

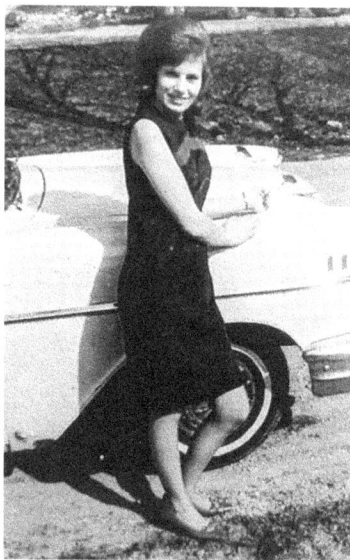

Dava leaning against Gary's '57 Chevy. (1966)

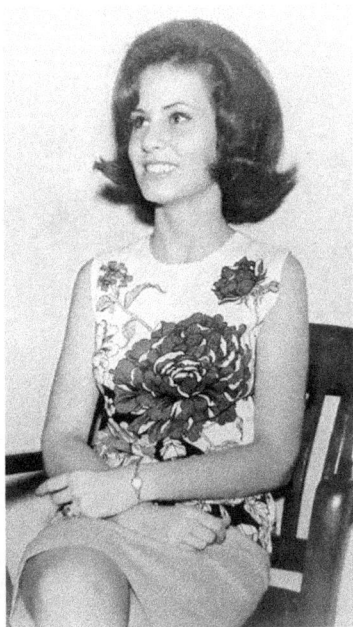

Dava working at a law office. We were engaged. (1967)

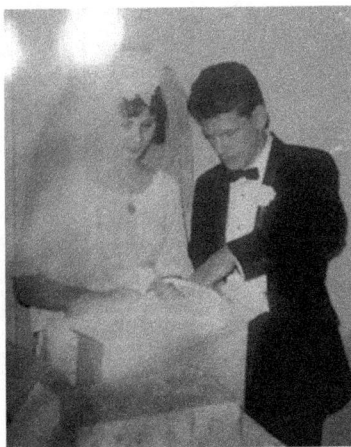

Dava and Gary Doyen's wedding reception. (1968)

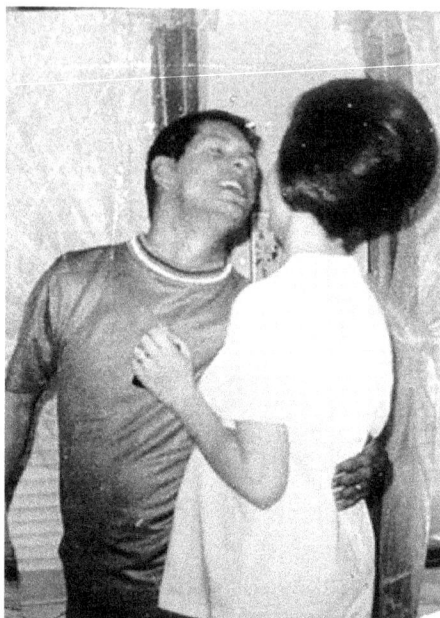

Dava and Gary two weeks before service in Vietnam. (May 1969)

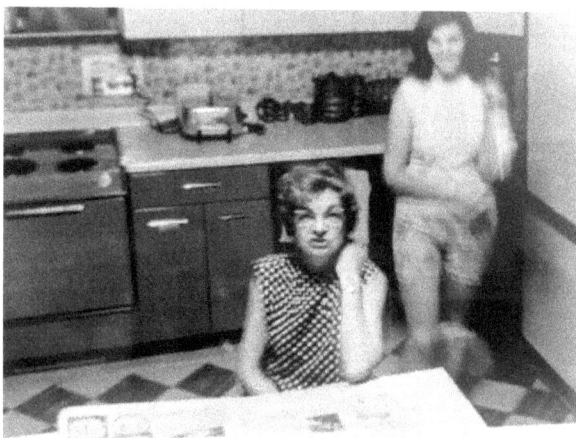

Dava with Gary's mother, Gwen Doyen. (1970)

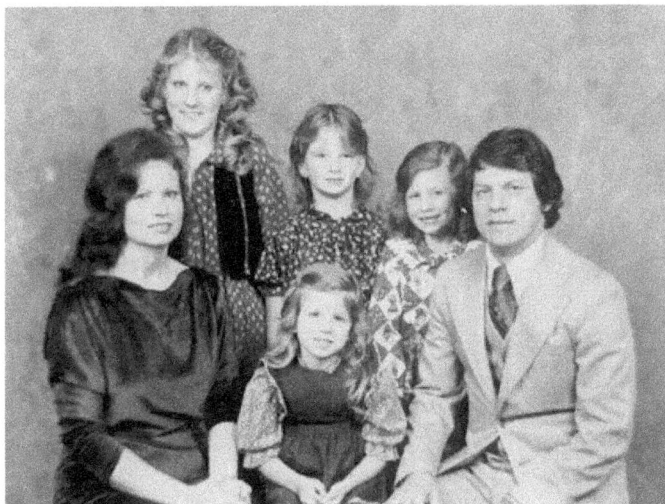

Dava and Gary with daughters Steph, Carrie, Andrea, and Sarah. (1982)

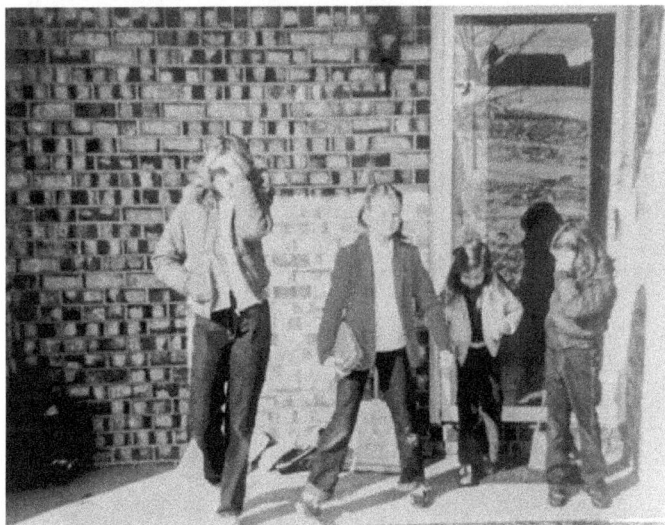

Our girls Steph, Carrie, Sarah, and Andrea. (1982)

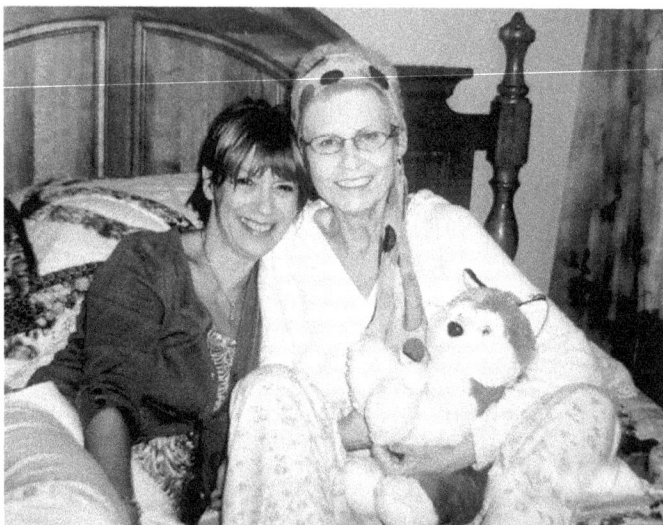

Dava and Judy on our 40th wedding anniversary. (2008)

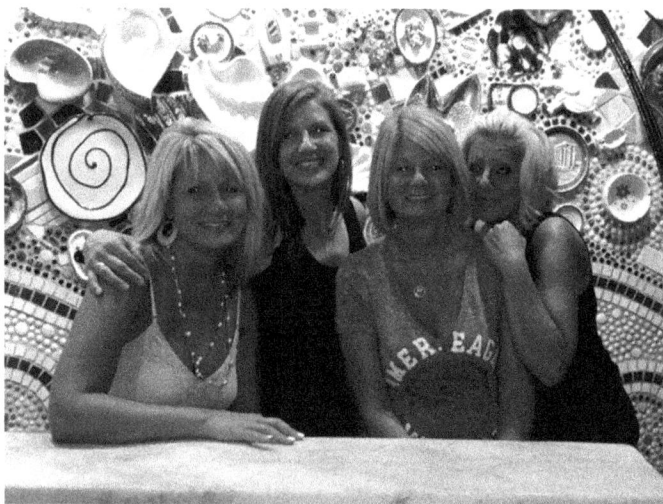

Daughters: Andrea, Sarah, Carrie, and Stephanie.

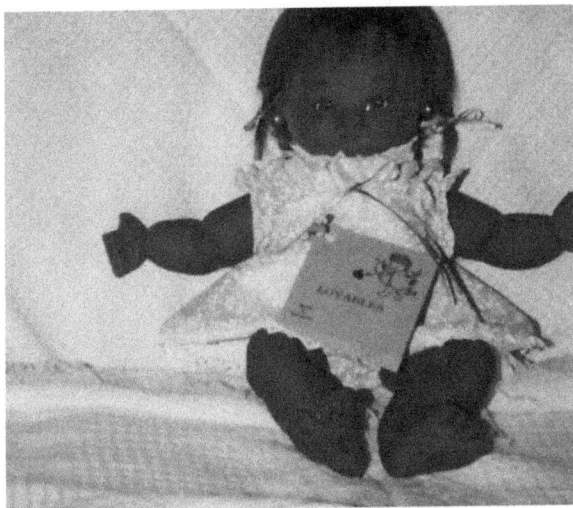

Doll made by Dava named Pearl.

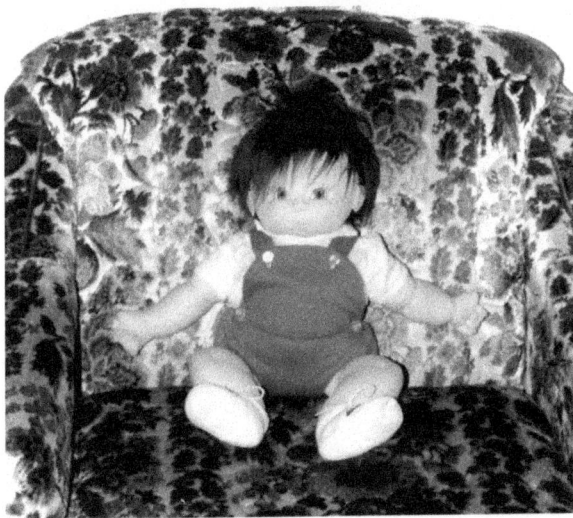

Doll made by Dava named Bartholomew Aloysius.

chapter thirteen

───────────── ∿ ─────────────

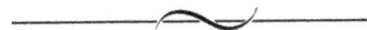

Thinking Destiny in the Dimness of Winter

As the days of winter roll by, it's easy to get caught up with the thought that this is the season of my life. When nature shows itself frozen in time, our minds drift into the abyss of stillness that only winter can bring. We think our time may soon be stilled as well. Though Dava was handling the treatments quite well, her mind was dealing with the inevitable truth. This is her January 25th entry:

I wonder what it feels like to die – I mean if in my case, when you feel almost ok, does it not feel anything physically? Will I just painlessly slip away not even realizing that it was an easy ending? Or will I have pain first or will it all be a rapid process? Shouldn't have watched "Love Story" last night.

It was truly a rare coincidence with Dava's diagnosis occurring on October 4, 2007, that on October 22nd of that same year, Oprah Winfrey had Randy Pausch as her guest.

He had been diagnosed with stage four pancreatic cancer nearly a year before and was known for his recent book, *The Last Lecture*. Dava and I watched the interview and realized he was one amazing individual. With a wife and three young children, he was facing the same prospects as Dava though he was twelve years younger at forty-seven years of age. Randy knew his fate, that he would not survive the disease, yet showed a remarkable courage along with his deep love for his family or anyone listening. He brought the dreadful cancer out in the spotlight that day for us to witness. Just hearing another person talk of the trials, pain, and aggressive nature of pancreatic cancer and bring it right into our presence while we were sitting in our living room was unexpected. We had heard someone who knew the rough road ahead, for he had been fighting it for months whereas for Dava, it was weeks.

In some ways, it had to scare Dava to know that this young man in his prime faced his situation with a sense of hope but also a realization that the odds were stacked against him. Having a recognizable face, a person we learned to know better, speaking so eloquently as to what matters most in life, made us feel that we had someone in Dava's corner who knew the struggle she was facing, and that was a measure of comfort. I can't remember if we bought his book, *The Last Lecture*, or where I read it, but I do know he taught me a valuable lesson that I have not forgotten. He was visiting his older sister and was preparing to take his nieces and nephew for a ride in his new car. His sister told the children they could not take their sodas and candy in his new car. Randy calmly said everything was fine and proceeded to empty the remaining contents of a can of soda on his car seat. We had already raised our kids, but with the grandkids, I started taking his lead and stopped letting things that might get in the way of sharing time with them, like worrying about a mess, bother me. That was probably minor compared to the strength and courage he showed that day on the *Oprah* show, and we had him to look up to when things were not going well. And Dava mentioned in her journal that *"a young man with pancreatic cancer was a guest on Oprah today."* The following morning she added, *"Didn't sleep a wink last night – all sorts of thoughts going thru my head – thinking mostly about the guy on Oprah's show w/pancreatic cancer."*

It was in the early part of 2008 when the news broke of Patrick Swayze's diagnosis of pancreatic cancer. Dava and our four daughters all enjoyed watching Swayze in *Dirty Dancing* and *Ghost*. Dava probably wouldn't confess it to me, but she *really, really* liked him as did millions of his fans. Again, we had someone to relate to, in this case a celebrity facing the same reality that Dava was facing.

The second person in three months' time who appeared so fit and healthy on the outside but did not have many options to prevent the cancer from taking over.

A few days after we heard the news about Swayze, I made a call to my sister Judy, a Disney vice president in California, and I asked her if there would be any way we could communicate with him. Judy told me she knew his agent from a previous occasion and would check to see if there was any possibility to relay our wishes. Within a few days, Judy returned my call to say that she had made contact with Swayze's agent who informed her that the family was keeping it a private matter at this time. I could understand their need for privacy, for he had just been diagnosed.

It wasn't that he was 'the movie star' that I wished for Dava to speak with him, although for Dava to hear from him would have been something my eyes would have loved to behold. I simply wanted her to speak to someone who had been dealt a similar hand. Later that week, I requested a list of names from the Lustgarten Foundation of people who were dealing with pancreatic cancer and were available to correspond. The list had twelve numbers, and I called all twelve. Dava was not sold on the idea. She thought these people had enough to deal with without our bothering them, but I was wanting to hear if anyone on the list was having any success with treatments or not. There was no initial response; so I, hoping to hear from one or more, left voice messages to each. Nearly ten days went by before a gentleman called on a Saturday evening and said he had received my message. He shared with me that his wife would definitely want to speak with my wife but that presently she was in the hospital. I conveyed my concern, and he said he would call when his wife returned from the hospital. After thanking him, I felt some excitement. Now I thought we could speak with someone who knew exactly what we were experiencing; however, I never received a call back. To this day, I have no idea what happened to that man's wife, and I wish I had asked him more questions at the time so as to have information to keep in touch. With pancreatic cancer, time is not on a person's side. Had she succumbed to the disease or was she too sick to share because there was no way for her to state the obvious, that she was in death's throes? I'll never know, but I guess Dava had sensed from the first that my efforts were much like a gladiator talking to another of his comrades just before his opponent killed him. Everyone in this arena especially is aware that death's escape door is as narrow as the gate that the camel passes through when entering the eye of the needle.

Sure, there is that glorious gift of hope that keeps the desire to be a survivor alive within one's being, and yet it's difficult for me to unfold the feelings that are so rampant regarding the helpless hope one feels when everything in the external universe is projecting an undeniable and dismal demise. Did I ever genuinely have the conviction that somehow nature's course would change? I still remember nights when all that entered my thoughts was a vacant side of the bed in the foreseeable future. Once outside on a Sunday afternoon on the driveway, I paused and looked at a window of our house as Dava was resting inside, and in a salient thought, said to myself that one day I will enter the house and Dava will not be there. Many times that moment has reappeared in my memory, but in that first instance, she was there. Why that moment suddenly came upon me I don't know, for I hadn't given up hope, that malleable, mysterious yearning called hope.

Snow had arrived on the first of February, and Dava requested that I take a picture of her statue of St. Francis of Assisi which was directly in her view outside the kitchen window. She was humored at the scene she had been viewing while standing at the sink. His beard of snow along with his head of white made for a simple and serene depiction of St. Francis, much in the way he was pictured in life. I noticed of late that Dava turned more toward heavenly inspirations than earthly yearnings that seemed less fruitful, though she still was very much into daily living, mainly because of her desire to be with her family and enjoy their presence. She wanted to do so many of the things she used to do, as the saying goes, in spades. But now even the simplest chores became somewhat of a burden due to her lack of energy.

In early February, Dava also completed her second journal book and noted that when she started her first one there was some doubt that she would live to begin a second, and yet she finished her second and began her third on February 9th. Many of her days' entries in the second journal began or ended with a scriptural quote or some provocative statement from other sources. Here is how Dava concluded one day's entry where she was writing about her dread of beginning another chemo treatment:

The Chinese have a way of saying what I need to do, 'You cannot stop the birds of worry from flying over your head, but you can prevent them from making a nest in your hair!' (I say, that depends on if you have any hair!)

It does my heart good to read such entries of this nature. Though she had a heavy burden to carry, she walked through the storm with courage and exemplified a lot of humanness throughout the ordeal. Dava was a person who let her feelings surface, and the journal let her express her fears, desires, humor, and above all, her love.

Dava at times acknowledged, when among me and the girls, the presence of a heavenly body almost casually, just mentioning that she peripherally glimpsed at eye level an angel pass near, but just as quickly, it passed as in a flash of light I presumed. She never made a major episode out of her experience, mainly just noting that one had passed by, and then she would continue a conversation or whatever she was occupied with at the time. Looking back on those few incidences, I think that's what made it seem a simple part of her journey; without any undo bluster, she calmly recognized a visitor whose realm her foot had begun to tread. I must say, as a witness to the few times the happenings occurred, obviously unaware until she spoke, it was the gentleness and casualness of her soft pronouncements that made me wonder. Dava was not what I would refer to as a religious seeker. She was fervent in her beliefs, but she never proselytized, and she never enjoyed being in an argument over religion; hers was a quiet one. And for certain, Dava would not want me deciphering her this way. She would be giving me that tight-lipped expression that tells me I am treading on thin ice. With that said, I do believe she was suddenly aware of something otherworldly, and her simple way of expressing that made a lasting impression.

Her journal entry of February 21st sort of sums up many of her nights: *It's about 12:15 am – I just don't feel good physically or emotionally. The thoughts that run thru one's mind can be so overwhelming.* The days were mainly taken up with working through her weekly chemo treatments. Every Tuesday since mid-October 2007, Dava had received Gemzar, pancreatic cancer's choice of chemo, and by Wednesday night, the effects began to wear on her. Most Thursdays and Fridays everything in her system seemed to be in reverse. Her food had no taste to it, and her bathroom schedule could go from extreme constipation one week to extreme diarrhea the next week. But it was the extreme fatigue that stayed with her usually until late Saturday, and by Sunday, she would begin to recover some of her energy. After a halfway restored, normal Monday, she had to once again contemplate her return for another chemo treatment on Tuesday to start the process all over again. This procedure was a constant with pancreatic cancer patients for the most part. The chemo had to be given weekly with never an end in sight.

Dava's journal entry of Sunday, March 2nd included this: *Tomorrow is my last good day before chemo on Tuesday.* So that Sunday, she must have started feeling somewhat better with Monday being what she called "one more good day." She was still having to take her daily Tarceva chemo pill each night, sometimes feeling nauseous, and with the pain in her back throbbing as a reminder that the tumor was fighting too, and this was what she considered her good day. One big constant that was never out of her orbit was the devastating thoughts that entered at will. Her journal entry on Thursday, March 6, 2008, serves as a good example of such thoughts:

"I don't feel well, my legs hurt and my back really hurts today and all the talk about Patrick Swayze's having pancreatic cancer has left me thinking about my situation. The report on him said that less than 4% live five years, and that most people die 3 to 6 months after diagnosis. Well, I'm 5 months into this awful thing – Oh Dear God, don't let me die yet. I need so much more time and so do my love ones, especially Gary and the girls."

The situation described here, and the grim statistics would worry any sound mind!

In the medical vernacular, a chemo session consisted of three straight Tuesdays of chemo with no chemo scheduled the fourth Tuesday so that Dava's blood counts could recoup. Then after two complete sessions, about eight weeks, a CT scan was performed to see how the progress was being maintained. Thus far the Gemzar chemo was doing its duty which was to keep the cancer at bay. For most of the winter season and the month of March, the cancer was growing at a slow rate, but the excruciating pain was there from the beginning. So even though the tumor was growing at a slower rate, the pain was actually increasing; no matter how slow the growth, the terrible pain was increasing relentlessly.

chapter fourteen

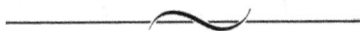

Spring Brought with It Radiation Treatments and More Hospital Stays

The month of March 2008 brought along an early Easter and a return visit from Dava's brother Scott and his family. It was an uplift for Dava to have her sibling travel to visit, for she had not been with him since our Thanksgiving gathering. Three of her siblings lived out of state, and therefore it was more difficult for them to see her on a regular basis, so Scott's arrival pleased her greatly. Our daughters, grandkids, and Dava's mom and dad all joined together with Dava and me and Scott's family for an afternoon Easter feast and festivities. Later that evening, Dava was able to share with Scott, her youngest brother, their family photos of times gone by; she very much enjoyed these echoes of earlier times. It was a good weekend all around; though the cancer and chemo tried to wear Dava down, they failed. Her spirits showed like the sun, for everyone in the house that day, the children, her parents, and her brother. They were of her blood ties; and I knew her love for me.

Paging through Dava's journal entries from the latter part of March reveals a definite escalation of her back pain, accompanied by other symptoms showing up as well. Her journal entry from March 24th, 2008, says, *"My nose and gums have been bleeding the last few days. I really believe my time is closer than I'm ready to accept."* She also mentioned that her urine was darker in color and that her stools had a grayish look. We later learned that it all had to do with the digestive system not performing properly since the pancreas controls so many of those functions, and it contained the cancerous tumor. But as April, the seventh month after her diagnosis, approached, it was positively the pain in her back and stomach that caused the greatest concern.

As noted earlier, Dava disliked the idea of taking pain pills, at least until the pain became unbearable. She reasoned it made her drowsy, and she wanted as much as possible to live through the daylight hours awake. Three lines, separate and distinct, from John Keats's "Ode to a Nightingale" stated a similar sentiment: "My heart aches and a drowsy numbness pains my sense // though the brain perplexes and retards // But here there is no light."

On the other hand, my solution was always that she should take the pain pills to counter the oncoming pain. Even though I tried to understand her position, how can anyone except the person who has gone through such an experience really know? I just wanted her to know that I hated to see her in so much pain. Then I brought up the subject of radiation again at supper with Mary Lee, Dava, and me present. Dava said she wished that I would stop suggesting radiation. Her journal entry, April 25th :

"Gary made me feel badly at the dinner table while Mary Lee was sitting with us. He just said, 'I will never bring it (radiation) up again. I will let it be the doctor's voice or let the Good Lord do what is necessary.' He almost looked angry, yet hurt, that I wasn't considering the treatment. I told him I wasn't unappreciative – that I was just scared."

That exchange certainly brings that night into focus, and I recall the discussion just as Dava recorded it in her journal. We had spent the previous Tuesday and Wednesday in the hospital because of the pain. There she was able to push the morphine button when the pain became too severe. As far as receiving radiation, it was her call to make, and I wasn't angry or hurt. I remembered the words from the renowned pancreatic surgeon that chemo followed by radiation might be the best solution to fight the tumors. Before being admitted to the hospital on Tuesday, Dava pleaded with Dr. Van Amburg to not send her home in the pain she was experiencing, and he then said he was admitting her. Looking back on this whole situation, knowing now so much more of both the good and bad, Dava was right in her assessment and fear of radiation on her system. I was jumping at anything I thought would give her relief, and I say as she had often said, *I'm sorry*.

There are just so few options to consider with this particular type of cancer. Its very nature is one that's extremely aggressive, even if the Gemzar performed as expected. The cancer seemed to fight that much harder for its own life's blood. On Tuesday, April 29th, Dava had her scheduled chemo session where she informed the doctor while being examined that her pain was still as severe as last week when he admitted her to the hospital. Dava's journal entry regarding this visit:

> *"Soon as I told him my back pain was still there he wanted us to talk to the radiologist oncologist Dr. Karen Halverson. Dr. Halverson said the radiation would help shrink the pancreas tumor as well as relieve the pain I'm having."*

During our conversation with Dr. Halverson, she covered most of what was included in the preparation and what might be expected out of the procedure. She stated that some patients had survived two years, and sometimes there was not much benefit. Finally, she added that the cancer *does return* but hopefully this treatment provides a somewhat better quality of life.

That evening Dava was feeling rather let down about the

visit in some ways. She mentioned the notion of two years as not nearly being the benefit she was hoping to hear, and I recall saying to her that we would take two years for now, then perhaps research will come up with something new in the future. Dava was wishing for ten years or twenty, not two; like the poet Keats who wished for ten years in order to express all his brain had to yield, she had every right to feel that way. In addition, she was so scared of what might happen within her system after this burning of bad cells along with the good cells ended. For the area of the body intended was indeed very sensitive to such extreme intrusions as the radiation would release on most of the main organs of her body. She had a reason to be scared more than I realized at the time.

She knew Dr. Van Amburg held off the radiation treatment for reasons he had expressed early on during our doctor visits. He had recanted a scenario where a patient's organs nearly turned to concrete. That was within the first month of Dava's treatments that he mentioned that case when I had inquired about the use of radiation, and Dava never forgot about that story. At the very least, she was worried that things were progressing much faster. The pain was increasing severely, and the Percocet pain pills wouldn't quench the constant, quivering pain. Dava's journal thoughts from that evening:

"Why I'm so afraid to die – Heaven is to be beautiful and

peaceful, but will I end up there, will I know those who have gone before me, why do I have to leave those I love here on earth – So many questions and no answers. Am I afraid of the pain in the end – will I have pain, or will I know if I have pain. Can those I leave carry on without me? – Of course they can – they are pretty much carrying on without my help – I want so badly to help the girls w/ the grandkids, I want so much to be with my parents, and I want so very much to love Gary more than ever. I just don't know what I'm doing – Father in Heaven, stay by my side and guide me to do what is right."

I feel it necessary to mention that our daughters and grandkids were in touch with their mom almost daily. Always one or two would come out for an hour or two and fix dinner or just bring the grandkids to visit their grandmother whom they loved, especially when she would ask one of the little ones to come sit by her. Any time I was away from the house, one of the girls would stay with her mother till I returned. There was just no way to reverse the situation that was in their midst, and only they could make their mother's pain either subside for an hour or at least keep her mind away from the pangs of pain. We did let them know that the doctors were planning to start radiation treatments to try to ease the pain.

The night before our Tuesday's doctor visit when Dava told the doctor she didn't want to go home until her pain was somewhat manageable, our daughters all came to the house. They were aware that their mom was having a very bad day, and one by one all four arrived, along with Kelsey, Carrie's daughter, in order to help her get through the evening any way they could. Dava's journal entry reads:

"Andrea had planned on being here, she brought KFC, but I wasn't able to eat. Carrie and Kelsey soon came out too, just to visit, not knowing how badly I felt. Pretty soon Stephanie showed up and then Sarah walked in my bedroom saying she couldn't be left out. They were all sitting on my bed while I was in the recliner. They reminded me of when they were all four little – Kelsey and Sarah even put on a wig show with my three lovely hair pieces. Then they all scurried around getting bags packed for Gary and me in case we had to go to the hospital before morning."

All I remember of that night was that those two hours they were all here were the best hours of that day for Dava, and that pleased me.

Dava sensed that the drastic increase of her back pain meant that the cancer tumor in her pancreas was letting her know it meant business. One night as we lay in bed, she suddenly spoke to me that she doubted if she would live to celebrate her July 17th birthday, her 60th. That was nearly three months away, but I quickly responded that there was no doubt she would celebrate her birthday followed by our anniversary in August. Her weight was holding up; her appetite on most days was sufficient, and her desire to live was forever present. Consequently, thoughts of the not too distant dates in the future became sort of a goal to reach. Seldom, if ever, was there talk of next year; however, we often did discuss the months ahead. Now her facing the radiation treatments became the main focus of our apprehensions, for what other choices were there? Dava's journal entry of May 1, 2008:

"Had such a good day yesterday until bedtime. My stomach was cramping and my back started hurting. I sat in the recliner in our bedroom and finally fell asleep – didn't wake till four in the morning. Got in bed and stayed there till seven. I have really been taking the pain pills – every three hours instead of the four prescribed – my pain isn't going away. The pills take the edge off a little, but I must sit up – lying down is excruciating."

Her back pain must have been beyond anything I could have comprehended, for the only severe, deadly pain I could recall was when for nine days I suffered through a ruptured appendix at age seventeen. That pain was so horrific; I have told the story often through the years to Dava's usual response, saying, "Oh no, not that story again." I probably came within a day of dying, and her pain at this point was more likely of a similar nature. I got relief after the ninth day after finally having emergency surgery, but Dava's prospects were that the situation would only become worse. At this juncture, I often prayed, "Oh Lord what doth lie in store for one with such suffering?" Dava's demeanor was a determination to fight with all her might through the pain, and for months of lonely nights, she had contemplated the trials ahead, and she braced herself to bravely face them. Here is another journal entry on the subject of her pain:

> *"My darn stomach is still hurting, and it is the weirdest feeling – a churning cramping, a grinding sort of feeling. I took a pain pill at 8 pm, another at 9 pm, my Tarceva chemo at 10, and I will probably have to take a sleeping pill at 11 – becoming a regular little junkie."*

On Saturday, May 3rd her back was still causing her considerable pain, but I think I was able to provide her with a distraction. Dava was always the fixer-upper all along, but now I needed to start what I had avoided most of our married lives, being the fixer-upper. Her journal entry that day:

> *"I watched Gary successfully hang the squirrel baffles on our bird feeder stands. He went out there after running on the treadmill, no shirt and sweating and then a bird shit on his arm – he was wiping his arm on the grass and finally came in and put a shirt on before going out – asking if I'd seen what*

happened – Oh I did with a laugh. He made the bed after taking a shower, straightened the bathroom, vacuumed the carpets, and put away the clean dishes and had fixed break-fast, gathered the trash and kissed me bye before going to check on the store. Now how many women out there can say they have even half that attention from their man. Yes, I know how lucky I am."

Well, I just simply could not resist putting this entry in here. I'm surprised the job of putting the baffles on the feeders went so well, despite the birds getting over excited and showing me no respect, or maybe they were delivering the message that it was about time *you* did something around here. In all honesty, I did manage to take care of the outside chores, like cutting the grass, raking the leaves, and any heavy moving, but when it came to repairing, or fixing something broken, Dava took the lead. Like I said before, she possessed the natural talent for fixing anything that needed fixing.

Dava's hair pieces were mentioned in one of her journal entries, and I had suggested one afternoon that we go to a Festus wig shop and just see what they had to offer. As soon as the sales lady realized that Dava had been through cancer treatment, she treated her royally. Dava tried on three and asked what I thought looked best. I suggested she take all three which were the same hair color as she had always had, a beautiful reddish, brown tinted piece. Her hair was still beautiful, but the chemo had thinned it a lot, yet when she combed in the hair piece, it was like, well, not many in her present condition could have looked any more beautiful. And Dava knew exactly how to weave her own hair into the wig to make it appear almost natural. She was happy, and that's what I wanted for her.

The very next night, Sunday, May 4th, Dava had a rough time. At bedtime, she was hurting and took her pain pills and Tarceva chemo pill which made her suddenly very nauseous. Her entry that night:

"About midnight I had a gripping pain in my stomach – I had just taken my pain pill and Tarceva before going to bed and just felt sick. Well, I threw up 'violently' – haven't thrown up like that since the week before my diagnosis."

I was really concerned, but she told me she felt better physically but was unsure why she suddenly got so sick. Something was not right.

The following Wednesday, Oprah had a few minutes of revisiting Randy Pausch who was dying from pancreatic cancer. He told Oprah he had kidney failure, congestive heart failure, and that his weight had dropped significantly the past several months. As we looked at the television screen, he didn't look good at all. He looked almost like my friend who came into the store in 2006 suffering through his final months of this disease. His cancer had for sure taken the upper hand. It was now only a matter of time before it would totally overtake him. As we watched, I thought: is this what's in store for us in the months ahead? Dava, however, was more concerned with his leaving his wife and children; that was in her nature to think of those who would feel his loss the most.

It was now May 14th, Dava's first of thirty-five radiation treatments. There were about twenty patients in the waiting area awaiting their time to be called for the treatment. The nurse at the receiving desk gave Dava a round pop sucker which contained morphine to suck on. She was the only patient I could see who was given that type of medication before treatment. She was in pain as she was most of the time, so I presumed it made it more probable that she could lie still while the radiation was being administered. She also took pills for nausea because there was a good chance she might get sick from the radiation bouncing off the pancreas which lies just below the stomach. Sure enough, after the thirty-minute treatment, we stopped by a Steak 'n Shake for lunch, and after Dava took one bite, she ran to the restroom to throw up. We then just left our food and headed home hoping this wasn't the script that we would be following for the next eight weeks. I was definitely beginning to realize the fears that had been running through her mind about radiation therapy.

After about eight days of radiation, Monday through

Friday each week, I noticed one other patient who was given a pop sucker while waiting her turn for treatment. An older lady was with her son as I discovered when I approached him and inquired as to what cancer she had. He informed me that she had pancreatic cancer. As the weeks passed, I thought to myself: of all the people in this waiting area over the eight weeks of radiation treatments, only two were given the morphine pop suckers, Dava and the older lady, and they both had pancreatic cancer. I am not suggesting that any of the patients were not suffering, for I'm sure some were, but most could converse and go in and come out seemingly unfazed, whereas Dava tended to get sick shortly after her treatment. It was the area of the body that made it so horrible.

Along with her scheduled radiation treatments, Dava also had to endure another type of chemo, referred to as Chemo 5FU, running through her body twenty-four seven. It was attached to her almost like a handbag, dripping chemo into her system constantly. The 5FU chemo was less toxic than the Gemzar and was part of the plan to keep all the cancer tumors somewhat in check. She was also still ingesting her Tarceva chemo pill each night before bedtime. A logical question could be asked: how does anyone exist with any sense of normalcy when so much poisonous material is spreading through one's body? It was quite obvious it wasn't good for Dava. She started losing her appetite and was often sick at her stomach. As a result, her weight began to drop, and much of the time, she was just miserable. She dealt with the feeling of being nauseous on a daily basis, and I know how I dread that feeling if it comes just once annually. To counter the nausea, she was having to take a number of prescriptions along with her pain meds. The doctors switched some of her pain pills in favor of a fentanyl patch, a potent pain reliever, to alleviate the nausea and improve her appetite. It was imperative for Dava to keep her food down in order to keep her from becoming too weak. She still had the will to fight through her misery, but she needed to be strong enough physically to put up the same fight as she had thus far.

On May 24th, Dava was again admitted to the hospital due to a combination of problems: severe back pain, weakness, nausea, and stomach cramps. The doctors thought there may even be a blockage in her intestines. It was difficult to determine exactly what the radiation effects were having on her. Each day in her journal, Dava listed at the top how many more treatments were left to complete the thirty-five scheduled, and I was equally anxious to count them down to zero like when we both were counting down the days when my Vietnam tour would end. It seemed at this point that the days could not pass fast enough. If the roles had been switched, I would have probably thrown in the towel, but Dava confronted the daily challenge with as much grace as humanly possible. When she got a little reprieve from the nausea, she would eat and describe in her journal the menu and how she managed to get the food down and keep it down.

The hospital stay lasted a whole week where her bowels were cleared using enemas, and she was able to keep her food down. On one of our trips from Dava's hospital room to take her radiation treatment, we had an experience that became a memorable one. It was early in her hospital stay with Dava in her hospital gown looking quite frail from all her sickness, and the room of patients was wall to wall. She was going to have to wait for nearly an hour before her turn. A precious lady went to the nurse's station and asked them to switch her position of order so that Dava could receive her treatments much sooner.

A nurse came over shortly after we were situated in the waiting room and informed us that Dava would be next in line and gave her the nausea medicine and morphine pop sucker. She said that one of the other patients had given Dava her slot in the rotation. I know my heart leaped a bit when the nurse relayed that message. When I asked the nurse who the person was, she pointed her out to me. I proceeded to thank the lady for her thoughtfulness, and she simply stated that she could see that Dava was in a weakened state and she wanted to help her. Bonnie was her name. From that time on, we always looked for Bonnie and her husband, and we got to know them as friends; the memory of her kind gesture would remain in my thoughts and memory forever. She didn't expect any praise and didn't want any; she just wanted to help. Bonnie's sacrifice of waiting that extra forty minutes for Dava's sake turned out to be a treasure of ten years for me.

About midweek of her hospital stay, Dava asked Dr. Busiek if she could have the 5 FU chemo discontinued. She told him that she didn't think she had the strength to do both radiation and the chemo. The doctor consulted with Dr. Van Amburg and decided to remove the 5 FU chemo. Dava and I were very pleased with the decision, for she just did not seem to have the stamina to continue both treatments.

As of June 9th, Dava had fourteen treatments remaining, and believe me when I say, this therapy was an all-consuming venture for the two months of the daily trips for treatment, the sickness, and the relentless, overall misery for Dava. The days of extreme nausea were frequent and would continue for the duration of the treatments. It is difficult to comprehend what those weeks were like unless one experienced them up close; for the one going through the process, it was pure hell. Just glancing at Dava's journal, I detected multiple days at a time when she wrote the simple statement, *"No entry, too sick."* On one day, she did write one sentence, *"Haven't felt like writing lately – haven't been able to keep my food down, have been dry-heaving and just feel terrible."*

I'm not sure, as I stated earlier, I could have endured the process of radiation: the feeling sick at my stomach for nearly three months, the throwing up and dry heaving, the pain, the anguish, the torture. Dava seemed to celebrate the few days when she didn't feel the pangs of the nausea and vomiting and even managed to give me her sweet smile when I did something for her. It remains an amazing reminder for me of her courage and strength under the duress of fighting the cancer and the treatments all thrown in her pathway, and yet she was able to smile.

That period in June also brought with it another hospital stay that lasted from June 6th to a noon release on the 11th. Again, it was mainly due to Dava's extreme sickness, weakness, and her being unable to keep her food down. There were still twelve more radiation treatments as of June 16th, and she had lost fifteen to twenty pounds already from the sessions. These last ten to twelve treatments might be compared to the dilemma a decathlon athlete faces who does nine very difficult events and then has to go all out to run the fastest mile of his life when his energy has been spent. The winner, however, sucks it up and makes it a sprint to the finish line to take first place and be awarded his gold medal. Dava needed the same endurance to reach the end of her radiation goal line, but there was no medal awaiting her, only a future of more challenges and adversities for each day the tumor progressed and grew, and the scans and blood work indicated worse results each time thereafter.

chapter fifteen

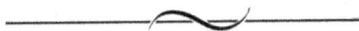

Our Long Journey Together Continues

Soon after Dava completed her thirty-fifth radiation treatment, she and I wanted to feel like she had conquered her enemy, for she was still standing, but we knew the stealthy tumor was lingering in wait to take advantage as soon as we let up even for one moment in this fight. As we sat together on the sofa contemplating the ups and downs the radiation treatments had presented to us, the mere fact that they were finished became our biggest highlight of the evening.

A channel on the television was broadcasting a concert, showcasing Robert Plant and Alison Krauss's new album, *Raising Sand*. Dava and I both enjoyed the songs they performed, and I mentioned that I wanted to purchase their CD the next time we went to the mall. Why was this important to mention in the situation we were in at the time? The following day one of the girls took her mom out shopping for a bit, and Dava bought the album for me. So again, what's the big deal having an album we both enjoyed? It was a few days later when I returned from a morning at the store that Dava asked me if I had listened to the last song on the CD. I told her I listened to six or seven songs but had not heard the last song. Dava then asked me to play the song "Your Long Journey" saying it seems to be our song. I put the song on and immediately discovered that she was absolutely right. It was so sad to hear the lyrics express what neither of us could ever bring ourselves to think much less say to one another. As we listened, we held each other's hands with tears filling our eyes; that was the only time we played that song until her funeral. It was just too painful.

I don't believe it was by coincidence that we rambled through channels until we landed on the concert, nor that Dava was the first to listen to the final song and present it to me as our story, our journey. I wasn't wanting to go where the words of the song were taking us, but in reality, it was happening to us. This duet, her to him and him to her, sung in the present, was the introduction to the day of our last goodbye.

My side of the family had begun having reunions every other year on the weekends before the Fourth of July for first, second, and third generations beginning in 1996. Before that we would all gather together a couple of weeks before Christmas for a few hours of visiting, feasting, and singing. For two of our reunions, 2000 and 2006, Dava played an integral part in making them memorable by making books for each of the eleven from the first generation, combining photographs of previous ancestors, poems, written contributions, copies of talks that were given, and much more. Like I said, she had the innate talent for performing such tasks with ease. In 2006, she made videos of the reunion to be shared with accompanied music. This was no simple task back then, but Dava made it look easy, and it made our reunion a much more memorable event.

In January 2008, our nephew Mike in Chicago announced that he and his family were going to host the family reunion in July. At the end of our invitation, he wrote a very empathetic note to Dava in which he said his thoughts and prayers were with her daily, and he hoped she would feel well enough to attend this year's reunion, but he understood completely that it depended on her health at that time. As the time was getting closer, I began searching my mind for something memorable to send to those attending. With Dava in the midst of radiation at the time and the toll it was taking on her, we knew we would not be able to make the trip to Chicago. Here is Dava's journal entry for the 15th of June:

"It's 2:30 am on Sunday – Gary is making us some tea – we can't sleep. He wants to read some poems we had written to

each other years earlier – in the 90's. He had written one to me and then I gave a reply. He has spent the last few afternoons thinking about what he could send to the reunion – poor guy – he looks so forward to these reunions and for his sake I wish he would go. Maybe he's afraid something will happen to me and he wouldn't be here to take care of me. He is really showing his love for me right now – hope he didn't have a dream or thoughts of worry while I was asleep."

There wasn't the least thought ever of my going to a reunion and leaving my love, and though sometimes she suggested I go, I truly don't think she ever wanted me to go. Besides, as I told her way back when, we are in this together as one in being; and wherever she was is where I wanted to be; and she knew that. Dava mentioned the poems we wrote to each other, and I want to include them here, mine to Dava and Dava's reply:

Dava's Love 8 – 97

When one's life is built around another
No treasured love say sister or brother
Comes close; few experience this I guess.
Understand! Departure means loneliness.

Is it that life for some requires more space
The givers love and takers show no trace.
The opposite of love is not hate, it's I not us
For love is concrete, everything else is dust.

For if the two are to become as one
Then everything should be given, not some.
At completion when it is said and done
All involved, including ourselves, have won.

Dava's Reply 9 -15 -97
For thirty years these golden rings
On our hands have kept us bound
We were given four daughters,
Oh, what a Blessed Sound!

One day soon it will just be
The two of us once more
When precious time will escort
Our love through Heaven's door.
d. doyen
(To my one and only love, Gary)

Our daughter, Andrea, unbeknownst to me till recently, had begun a journal of her own in the late spring of 2008 during her mother's illness. Her first entry was May 23rd:

"Someone told me to start this journal, Mona Branson, mine and Mom's hairdresser – to save the memories of my Mom. Mona had lost her dad just months before w/ the same cancer as Mom, pancreatic; can hardly spell it, have no idea what part of one's body it belongs or what it does. All I know was

on Oct. 4th of 2007 I got a phone call from dad. Mom had been having a lot of back pain, the pain never went away. The doctor ordered tests – all the doctor said was "something" up with her pancreas.

"Now 7 months and 19 days later my Mom is sick everyday – she did about 22 chemo treatments and started radiation this week. She's having chemo every Tuesday for an hour each time, by Friday she is so sick. She begins to feel better and it's time to start all over again. The chemo didn't shrink her tumor, it just didn't grow as fast, – I guess that's good. Now w/radiation she is even sicker, it's so sad. She throws up going and coming to the hospital. She hardly eats, I think she has lost 25 lbs.

"I try to see her as much as I can between work and kids, I think she enjoys having us around. Just last night she asked me to shave her head. I asked if she was sure, she said her head itched and she wanted it gone. She sat in the wooden chair in the front hallway – off came her wig as she instructed me on how to use the clippers, repeating several times to go up, not down and begging not to cut her. I had tears in my eyes, but didn't let her see – I asked if she was sad, she said no, I told her I was. She has snow white hair, what's left anyway – nothing like the brunette or redhead she's been my entire life. She looks so weak, so much in pain, she shivers non-stop the whole time I'm clipping away. She's always so cold. She complains of her back hurting and that she is hungry – but knows it won't stay down. She lays on the sofa and keeps dozing off w/her mouth wide open, and actually looks somewhat peaceful. I get up to leave and kiss her eye, she tells me it was so sweet that she'll never wipe it off. I love her. I hate seeing her in this pain and often wonder if she'll be here this time next year. And the thought scares me. I can't imagine her not being here.

"And dad, I feel sorry for him – he has stayed w/her around the clock. He takes her everyday to St. Luke's and anywhere she wants to go afterward if she's up to it. When she can't sleep he watches TV w/her in the middle of the night – sometimes not going to sleep for 24 hours. He tries to cook if one of us can't be there, he asked me last night to boil eggs and took notes. He cleans the house. I see him always doing dishes. He worries mostly about Mom, it's sad. You do see true love there, I know I do – he has seen her at her worst – she throws up in the jeep everyday, sometimes she complains, and yet when I was shaving her hair off he told her how nice she looked – that's love. What did she do to deserve this – she doesn't smoke, drink, does nothing wrong – why my Mom? If I lose my Mom a big part of me will go w/ her – – I'm going to bed – goodnight Mom. I love you."

Andrea's May 24th, 2008 journal entry:

"Just got home from the hospital. Mom was very sick this morning when I called. Her back pain was the worst it's been, *she threw up all night and most of today. She said she wanted to die today. It's the cancer that is making her hurt so bad, the doctors had her on morphine. It's the radiation, next week it will be the same. I can't lose my time w/Mom. I don't want to regret not going that one day I needed to be there. I think the kids will one day understand. I would have taken them, but it would have saddened them or scared them to see their Granny like this. I can already see Emily backing off, not getting as close to her Granny as before. Not kissing her like she did, not eating after her. We were supposed to spend the night w/her – guess there is always tomorrow – did I just say that?"*

Andrea's May 25th, 2008 journal entry:

"Nope, Mom had another bad day, throwing up and back pain. Dad said not to come up, Mom pushed the morphine button every 30 minutes & got no sleep, nor did dad. The doctor loaded Mom up on drugs to help her sleep. I'm at my chapel hour right now – it's so peaceful in here – though it's storming outside and dark. I have no fear. I know God is watching over our family and He knows how strong our love is – I don't ever ask God why He did this to Mom, all I ask is that when the pain gets too much for her, please let her go. I know Mom, like my sisters & I don't want her to leave and can't imagine her not in our lives – but she'll be more comfortable in heaven. And if and when the time comes, I will let Mom know that we and the kids will be ok, and we will all

help Dad. No one knows this feeling of seeing your Mom in so much pain & scared to death – she may not be here tomorrow. You have no idea until you've been thru it & it sucks big time."

Andrea's journal entry on June 8th, 2008:

"My dear friend Linda rear ended a car and over corrected & hit someone head-on. I believe she died right away. It still hasn't sunk in with me, seems very surreal. She was the first person in De Soto to show me around town when I was 18. Tomorrow is her memorial – will be another sad day. Mom looked & sounded very sick today – so frail. I try to hold back my tears & stay strong. Her body can't possibly take 19 more radiation treatments – there's no way, but she'll die trying.

"For my last fifteen minutes in chapel I will pray for my Mom and friend. Please help Mom get through this awful disease and make her well & please help Linda's family. Goodnight Mom and goodnight Linda!"

Our daughter, Andrea, came out one Sunday in mid-June to visit with us and brought some food along with some lotions for Mom. As we three sat in the living room chatting, Dava, without much warning, told me to get the bucket because she had to throw up. I stood before her holding the bucket as she emptied her stomach. As I started for the bathroom to wash out the bucket, Dava called out that she needed the bucket again, so I held it as she vomited a second time. So there is nothing heroic about assisting the one you love by doing what I just did, but Andrea was well aware that whenever she or her sisters had a stomach virus, it was their mother who usually cleaned up the mess without any fanfare. Of course once or twice I tried doing my part to help; but after gagging and holding my nose, Dava would take over. What made this day so memorable to me was Andrea's Father's Day card the following Sunday. It read in part, "I knew how you were never able to clean up after one of us threw up and yet you were able to help Mom without any sense you were concerned about what you were having to do. I love how you love Mom." Her observation was correct. I felt so much love and compassion for her mother at that moment that I didn't have time for my quirks to act upon me.

Andrea's journal entry on June 22nd, 2008:

"Went to see Mom today, John and Onie had been there most of the afternoon. She had gone 24 hrs. w/out getting sick – and within an hour of being there she got sick. It's hard seeing her that way. I took Mom to radiation therapy on Wednesday with Carrie coming along. She came out feeling like shit, Three people walked her out – fanning her with wet clothes on her. They gave her two bags of fluids, she's just so weak. She still wanted to go shopping at Sam's. She bought lots of fruits. Got home and made her an egg sandwich and dad hamburgers. He loved them – boy is he picky! Dad called later

that evening & said that Mom was sick that evening. It's just not right for her to be so sick & in pain."

Andrea's journal entry on June 29th, 2008:

"I'm at my chapel hour again. It's always so peaceful here, not a sound. Mom has been in the hospital four days until her radiation was finished, went to her Friday when she got home, and she looks so weak. She gets a month of doing nothing – maybe next week she'll be Mom again and Dad can be dad again. – Going to Chicago for the family reunion Friday morning."

The radiation therapy came to an end on June 30th, and we didn't even celebrate, for it was like fighting a battle in Vietnam. So relieved that it's over and grateful to still be in one piece, one just wants rest and repose. Dava often told me how much she enjoyed making entries of her journey in her journal, and yet from June 17th through July 12th, there are no entries at all. That's how devastating the radiation therapy had been on her.

While most of the family attended the reunion in Chicago, Dava was going through the roughest period of her life to this point. My nephew Mike had arranged for a Skype type of connection for Dava and me to talk and share with everyone at the reunion on Saturday, July 5th, but that day Dava was so miserable, she could hardly lift her head from the pillow without becoming ill. So we canceled the filming part of the plans, and I placed a phone call to thank them for making the attempt but informed them that Dava was experiencing a very difficult evening. She and I were hoping that after the radiation treatments ended, she would be beyond all the sickness in her stomach, but we were later informed that it could take two to three weeks for the effects of the radiation to leave her body. So the two months of agony had turned into three months.

Andrea's journal entry on July 6th, 2008:

"Just returned from reunion in Chicago. Mike and Anne's house was huge & and beautiful – food, music, Mass – it was all nice. Felt a little different without Dad, Ralph, Pat, & Rob there – they must be the ones that keep the party going – seemed more quiet, laid back, but still very loud. Mom has been really sick all weekend, she's in an awful mood. But I wonder what mood I'd be in if I had this cancer and saw no good happening? I feel so bad for her. When will she get better or will she get better? I hope she doesn't go anytime soon, it's not good timing. We need her. She doesn't deserve this. I guess no one does, I'm not ready for her to go."

Dava's mom and dad were so good to call or email, and they came to see her nearly every Monday of every week of her illness. During this very trying time, they arrived one morning around eleven o'clock to find Dava lying on her bed and not feeling well at all. She was very restless with silent sighs escaping through her lips. Her mom immediately sat next to her and rubbed her hand, and her dad stood back and was shaking his head. In his quiet but firm way, he said to me that she might not have much longer to go on like this. I assured them that much of her misery this morning was stomach cramping and that her overall sick feeling was partially due to the doubling of her Ativan medicine which was supposed to relieve her nausea. I let them know that yesterday was a decent day for Dava and hopefully this bout of sickness would pass soon. After twenty to thirty minutes, her sick feeling subsided, and she was able to come to the living room to say that she felt somewhat normal. Sometimes these periods of extreme duress would hit and make her so sick. I understood that someone witnessing such severity of misery for the first time would be very concerned about the coming days. Later on in the day, Dava managed to eat one good meal which made the day less stressful for her parents.

A few days had passed, and Dava had another day like the one on Monday, so I called the doctor's office and was told she needed to be admitted to the hospital. After settling in at the hospital, Dr. Busiek, who practiced in the same office with Dr. Van Amburg, was making the rounds. As he talked with us about Dava's condition, she asked him if there was an estimated time of survival in her case in particular. Dr. Busiek began his answer by telling Dava that if she were attending college, she would have already graduated and been in the Masters program. That's how far she had already come through this disease. He was gentle in his comparative skills, but basically it meant that she was already on borrowed time and exceeding the norm for pancreatic patients by months. He wanted an ultrasound to be done because Dava was still having back pain and was often very sick. The ultrasound did not look at all positive, so he then ordered a CT scan which was scheduled for the next Saturday.

On Sunday just after the noon hour, Dr. Busiek came to her room and sat on the edge of the bed and said there was a "mixed bag" of news he wanted to share with us. The scan revealed that the liver had three more small tumors, and the lungs had several as well. He noted that the pancreas tumor had been damaged at its core with plenty of dead cancer cells. My first reaction to the news of more tumors on the liver and now some on the lungs was more of a frightful nature; even if the pancreas tumor was damaged by the radiation, it did not seem like a fair trade off. The doctor further explained how the nature of this type of cancer is very aggressive and that the continued use of chemo would hopefully keep the tumors in check. Dr. Busiek was a very compassionate man, and his connection with knowing my sister Judy in high school just added to his wish to make this "mixed bag" of information come to us as gentle and yet as direct as he could make it. Dava's journal entry that evening reads:

"I want so to remain here for all my children, my loving and caring husband, Mom and Dad and my family, but it looks like Jesus may have other plans for me."

From the hospital room that Sunday, soon after the doctor left us, I called all four of the girls and told them about the "mixed bag" of news. They all seemed devastated by the news about the newly discovered tumors. Sarah called her mom at the hospital and said her day was just not going right after she received our phone call. The radiation did its job of killing some of the pancreas tumor cells, but by Dava's not being on chemo, allowed the liver tumor to thrive and gain ground. I, personally, thought it was a bad trade off too, especially with all the horrible side effects the radiation had caused. The only positive result was that her back pain was somewhat diminished from its previous pulsating state, the reason given for starting the radiation. So on Monday we left the hospital to head home, it was definitely a day filled with a lot of mixed emotions; but Dava was having a fairly good day with no sick feelings and managing her pain with the pain patch and pain pills.

Andrea's journal entry on July 14, 2008:

"Mom's been in the hospital since Monday – a week tomorrow. Got awful news today – the doctor did a scan a month

early to see why she was hurting so bad, the tumor on her pancreas seems to be dying from the inside out – but they found 4 new tumors on her liver and more in her lungs. When Dad called, he surprisingly seemed cheerful & positive. I think that was for me, he was trying to hide his true feelings. Me I'm ticked, sad, frustrated, scared all in one. Seeing her today and knowing the cancer is only growing more makes it hard to believe she'll be here for Christmas.

"She'll go back to chemo Tuesday, doctors say that may extend her life – I know dying is a part of life, but I beg God not to let her go – no time is a good time – but she needs to see our kids grow, and they need her. She was so happy seeing them today. She pulled them into her bed the minute they walked in. She comes home tomorrow – I'll take the kids out, we'll have BLT's or tacos – whatever she wants. And I promised I'd paint her toes – she asked me in the hospital again today.

"I don't want Mom to suffer anymore. I know it's in God's hands – – I just can't imagine her not being around."

Dava's entry on July 17, her 60th birthday:

"Today is my 60th birthday! Who would have thought that a little baby girl born sixty years ago would have four beautiful daughters, four lovely granddaughters, and three handsome grandsons and the best husband ever!"

Another entry on the same day, July 17th:

"Judy's friend Jenny sent me a pretty lounging outfit yesterday – not necessarily for my birthday – just a thinking of you gift. How sweet – I don't know that I would ever think to send someone my best friend knew a gift to make her feel better.

Mary Lee asked Dava what she would like for her birthday dinner. She answered, *"pork steaks,"* so that's what we all had along with all the fixings, and brother Charlie brought a carrot cake. All the girls and grandkids were out that day too, and that was just what Dava needed, a good day all around.

Dava had her weekly doctor's visit on the 22nd, and Dr. Van Amburg gave her a little positive news that the tumors were small and that there would not be a chemo this week but would start a new session next week. On the following Saturday, we heard the sad news that Randy Pausch had died yesterday from pancreatic cancer. When one has the same, exact illness confronting her or him, that kind of news hits where it hurts. Again, Dava felt sad for his wife and children, but for both of us he was a heroic example of character, selflessness, and courage. We were both very sad that day to hear such news.

Dava's entry in her journal for August 2nd says, *"Happy Anniversary to us – 40 years."* Yes, we were married August 2, 1968. I was twenty-two years of age and Dava was a gorgeous twenty-year-old. Never did I envision the circumstances that now faced us. In fact, I thought in my old age if I ever needed a caregiver, Dava would be the first person in the whole world I would want in that role. So with my whole soul, mind, and body, I wanted to be there for her, and I'm sure I could never be as good as she; my desire and only wish was to be there with my love.

Judy came from California for the sole purpose of being with Dava and me for a few days. She had been a bridesmaid for Dava in our wedding, and they both enjoyed reminiscing through the pages of our wedding album. During her stay, I took some photos of the two of them and Dava writes:

"Then Gary took a picture of Judy and me with the outfit her friend got me – then he took a picture of Judy and me on our bed holding Jack, the stuffed dog Judy's friend Jackie sent me for my birthday. I'm wearing the outfit another of Judy's friends, Jennie sent me."

Photography is not one of my hobbies, but the picture of Judy and Dava on the bed was so good that I had it made into an 8x10, and it's hanging where it has been even while Dava was still with us. The camera date in the lower, right hand corner reads August 2, 2008. Dava was ten months into her journey and beautiful as ever.

Judy stayed from August 2nd to August 5th and spent two nights with us. She fixed meals and kept the kitchen spotless, but mainly she just shared her time with us and then headed back to Los Angeles. Also early in August my brother Jim came to visit from California. Dava thought the world of Jim, for he was so thoughtful and good to her. We had a lot of laughs along with some serious conversations and finished off the evening eating some Imo's pizza with Jim and Mary Lee.

On August 12th, we traveled to our weekly Tuesday's doctor appointment and Gemzar chemo session. Dava's blood counts were too low for chemo, so Dr. Van Amburg said we should wait another week and then resume treatments. We also had our final meeting with Dr. Halverson from radiology. Dava's entry after our meeting with her:

"She asked if we had any questions. Gary asked about the dead cells in the pancreas tumor that showed on the CT scan on July 11th. She said the tumor was still the same size, however, the center was fluid filled with dead cells, and that white blood cells were eating away the dead cells. My liver now has more tumors as does my lungs, all small now! Dr. Halverson thought that the radiation had done its job in attacking the pancreas tumor, but I still and will always remember her first words to me, 'the cancer always returns.'"

As time progressed toward mid-August and beyond to September, it was evident that Dava's overall condition was getting worse. After a few hours with our girls at the mall, she entered in her journal:

"When I got home I didn't feel well – had a slight temperature of 100.3 – if it gets to 101 we have to call the doctor. My ribcage feels so bruised. It all scares me so. I'll take my Tarceva at 10 pm, Lortab, and will try not to worry too much."

Then on August 11th she adds more on her condition:

"In the beginning they said my pancreas tumor was inoperable, incurable, and that treatments are to give me a better quality of life, but if there is still extreme pain, nausea and I don't have enough energy to be of any help to the children or Gary then why am I going through all this turmoil? I don't know if I want to continue with chemo – I'm just now beginning to feel halfway decent and after another treatment I'll be tired toward the later part of the week only to find out there are more tumors showing up. It's hard to keep fighting when you know 'the cancer always ultimately returns.'"

We did make the next Tuesday trip to begin another chemo session. Dava made a gift bag with pretzels to give to the nurse's station in the radiology department. Her entry reads:

"Wanting to take them a small gift of appreciation, they were so good to give me handfuls of pretzels when I was too sick to hold my head up. However, I don't know if my stomach can face another trip into that department again."

Knowing the circumstances concerning her illness were

becoming more and more challenging every day, it was amazing what the smallest ray of hope can bring about in one's life. On August 20th, Debbie called from St. Luke's and informed Dava that her cancer marker dropped to 29. Statistically that meant the cancer was not producing cancer cells, but realistically it meant it's time to celebrate. Again, she and I knew that in actuality the cancer marker news only meant a possible pause in cancer cell production at that particular hour, but there weren't too many occasions to feel excited about, especially with the news we had been receiving of late. I wanted this little window of hope for a few hours. Dava's entry after the phone call: *"Gary was so excited he made four phone calls, then told me to get my "pants on" – we are going somewhere even if it's Walmart."*

Well, that was a short-lived celebration, for on August 26th Dava was getting her regular Tuesday dose of chemo. Shortly after the treatment she recorded in her journal:

"I've felt flu-achy all over ever since I got chemo today. I took a pain pill around 4:45 – so far not much relief – it's now 6:32. I wish I could feel good so I would stop complaining and stop finding fault with everything. They say people with pancreatic cancer are unhappy – I believe it – but why? Is it because most of us have been diagnosed as inoperable or is it because we feel so miserable most of the time and can't feel any sense of happiness?"

Once the radiation was out of her system and the sickness subsided for a time, one would think better days may lie ahead after the grueling, past three months Dava endured. But the toll it took on her body, the three months of unrelenting sickness was evident. Dava writes, *"I'm dressed to go somewhere – all my clothes just hang on me – it's hard to believe how hard I used to try to lose weight to wear these clothes and now they are too big without trying."*

There were just so many days now that Dava was too tired or the pain too severe to make any plans for the week in advance or even for a day. It all depended on how she was able to cope at any particular time. The most effective way to reveal this period in our journey is again to use a few days of her own words from her journal. Her entry on September 5th:

"Gary and I drove to Fenton to Barnes and Noble, but I got so tired very very quickly, so we left and went to a Mexican restaurant where I ordered something then couldn't eat it, so we came home – should have just stayed home to begin with."

She then writes on September 11th:

"I haven't felt all that well lately – my bones feel like they're crushing from my neck to my hips. Guess I'll lie down for a while – I am aching all over. Gary tried to get me to eat an egg but I just didn't want it – he tries so hard and I make it so hard for him – pain does that."

She actually never made it hard for me. Throughout this our journey she bore most of her physical and mental anguish and torture alone, within her gracious being. I usually had to ask how the pain in her back was because I knew the positions she took to try to gain some relief. Dava used the quiet moments, usually in the early morning hours, to prepare herself for what lay ahead. It was truly amazing the amount of fortitude that emanated from her frail, gracious, and beautiful frame.

chapter sixteen

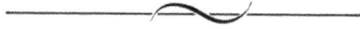

Reality Sets In

The date of September 16th has become one of those dates for me that makes one pause and reflect on how someone else had to face a rough day while the rest of the world was going about its business. On this date, Dava made an entry in her journal detailing how she wanted to be laid out for her visitation at the funeral home. As I related to her early on, I wasn't going to read anything she wrote in her journal as she wrote, but she did share segments with our daughters, and it became apparent later on that she had shared this entry to one or more of them. The entry reads:

> "If anyone gets this far reading my journal please know, as morbid as it seems, that I would like to be laid out in the end in a light blue jacket (suit jacket or light blue suit) make sure my make-up is on lightly, no base, just a tad of mascara, lip liner (light color liner) and a touch of blush. And please make sure my hair is not sticking up like Harpo Marx! Don't really

think I need my glasses on, and do not put my diamond wedding rings on me – So much for that! I love you. PS Changed my mind – want to wear grape colored suit I have if it still fits."

Dava even made a reference to this September 16th date at the beginning of her first journal. The 16th was on a Tuesday that she had received her chemo, and the doctor gave us some critical numbers concerning her blood tests, mainly with reference to the liver function. Of course, the liver is one of those organs that is indispensable to survival. When its function is hampered, it throws everything out of sync. Maybe this news caused Dava to make that entry on the evening of September 16th. She didn't mention any of these specific wishes to me, and I don't recall what I was contemplating that day; but I do know it wasn't anything like what she was thinking. She also added a touch of humor in something so serious. For me, it is just sad to read what was going on in her mind that night. It makes me want to go back and embrace her. We had talked of general things she didn't want at her funeral home visitation, like her saying she didn't want people standing over her saying she was now in a better place or other similar clichés.

There were two weeks in September when Dava did not write in her journal which was a warning that her system was becoming weaker and weaker. One night as we lay in bed in the darkened room, she spoke to me of her doubts that she would not be here for Thanksgiving. Though she had much less stamina, she had the resourcefulness for making the most of Mary Lee's stew or her good eating habit of eating fruits and drinking nourishing shakes. She still possessed the relentless will to fight this foe at every turn which gave me the determination to assure her we would celebrate Thanksgiving together. But as October approached, the anniversary of Dava's diagnosis, it was evident that she had her doubts as she writes in her journal:

"It's a beautiful fall day – I've been full of energy – well at least more than usual. This Autumn weather is so pretty one cannot truly appreciate its beauty until you're afraid of not seeing it again."

I'm sure John Keats, facing a similar fate, packaged all human feelings of living and dying into his ode, "To Autumn." Imagine living your life as if this is truly your last days on this beautiful earth. Dava kept most of such thoughts to herself and her journal, but we would talk about how things might evolve in the future, and I always tried to bring a positive scenario to our discussion, not unrealistic cures but more like tomorrow may be a better day. We both realized the eventual outcome, but why dwell on that instead of taking in and treasuring the precious time remaining, however long it was to be.

In the middle of October 2008, Dava said she would like

to spend a weekend with her mom and dad. I wanted her parents to have some time alone to share with their daughter unless she insisted that I come along. So on Saturday morning, the 18th, we drove down to Farmington where her parents met us. We visited for a few minutes before I hugged and kissed Dava goodbye and told her how much I loved her and to call me if she needed anything. This was the very first time since her diagnosis that I wouldn't spend the night with Dava, even during her hospital stays. She was wanting to have individual time with her mom and dad, and I was just hoping for her to have a wonderful weekend.

On Saturday night she called, and we talked about all the shops she and her parents visited and where they dined. She also said she missed me, and I asked if she wanted me to drive down, but she said it was only one more day and that we would see each other on Monday morning. She did sound happy to be with her parents. On the other hand, I had that heart wrenching feeling of total emptiness inside me. I felt like my mind was playing tricks on me all through the night, as though it was telling me what my future would be like without Dava. I sat quietly in the living room, no music, no television, and the tears began to flow. I knew that I needed her so much more than she needed me. I couldn't make it forty-eight hours without her, so how was I to face the future?

On Sunday, the 19th in the early afternoon, Dava's dad called to say that Dava had gotten sick and wanted to go home. I told him I would leave immediately to meet him in Farmington. I started feeling guilty because I wasn't there when she needed me, as if I could have done any more than her parents did for her. No, but I needed to have my arms around her when sickness got a hold of her. It took thirty minutes, and Dava and her parents were there waiting on me. Dava looked a little frail, but we hugged, and I knew then that I would never leave her sight for another night. Dava's journal entry of her visit :

"I did spend the weekend of Oct. 18 & 19th w/ Mom and Dad. Had a good time – we went shopping at Big Lots, Green's, Walmart, Value City, and Goodwill, all places Gary never likes to go. But Sunday, the 19th we ate at White Castle, which I was craving, then shopped at Walgreens, when I violently threw up in the car – Dad quickly gave me his Walgreen bag, so I emptied my guts into it, good thing there wasn't a hole in it."

The incident left me with more mixed emotions. First, I felt bad about not being there for Dava at that moment she became ill although the purpose of her visit was to have time to share with her parents. Secondly, after getting over the sudden sadness of her getting sick and hearing that she wanted to come home, I felt my heart swell with an abundance of love for her. So it ended up being just one night, one very lonely Saturday night. It was difficult to know who needed each other more. I didn't leave her side for even one night afterward, except when she was in ICU, and then I was able to stay in the waiting area and sleep on a sofa.

It happens that sometimes with diseases like pancreatic cancer there is insufficient time to come to terms with the finality the loved ones face for the one they love. There were two local cases of this type of cancer that approximated Dava's diagnosis, and both survived less than four months, having chosen to forgo treatments. Dava had just passed the one-year date since the October 4th diagnosis, and we had no idea at this point how many more months the battle could be fought successfully. We were indeed thankful for the time granted to us so far and for the chemo's effectiveness in keeping the liver tumors at bay for so long a period. However, as autumn progressed into October, I could sense that Dava's condition was getting worse. Her appetite was nearly gone due to her stomach sickness, and her stamina was failing fast causing her to spend longer stays lying in bed. Dava's mid-October entry:

"I look so thin – I can't understand the people who are anorexic and don't see themselves that way. I weigh the same or less as I did when I got married & at my age now I look like a scarecrow! Oh well, it is almost Halloween."

I'm sure Dava realized how her system was becoming weaker by the day. Then one night as we lay in our bed, she mentioned in no uncertain terms, that she wanted to know where she was going to be buried. At first, I replied something like it will work out when the time comes, but she repeated, "No, I want to know where I'll be." So I suggested calling Cathy Roop, a close family friend and a member of the Calvary Cemetery Board, and I asked Dava if I should inquire about an area with six plots; but she said she only wanted plots for her and me.

The following morning, I called Cathy, so she could meet with us later in the week. As Cathy searched the cemetery map locations, she noticed there were four unused plots beside my mom's and dad's graves. She contacted Mary Lee who had the deeds to the four plots, and my sister called me to see if Dava and I would be interested in two of those. After talking with Mary Lee again the next evening, I informed Dava that we could have the two plots next to my parents and that she would lie next to my mom. My mother was the last family member to have passed in 1976, and Dava was the last person to see her alive before she passed away from congestive heart failure. As soon as I mentioned that she would lie next to my mom, she said, "Okay," and she never spoke another word about it. I was not for certain why Dava was so adamant about where she would be buried, but it makes sense to me now. She was very organized and considered her burial place part of planning her life to the end. It is also comforting to me to know the location of my final resting place. At first, it was awkward for me to discuss Dava's burial place, but I am glad she did bring it up because it couldn't have worked out any better. On one journal entry in October Dava records:

"The Autumn weather is so pretty – one cannot appreciate its beauty until you're afraid of not seeing it again. – I've been in bed the last 3 days and ½ of today. Gary called Dr. Van Amburg and told him I had been running a low grade fever and that my urine has been dark. The doctor didn't seem too concerned, told me to drink lots of fluids. My appetite hasn't been good until last night when Mary Lee sent over some of her beef stew and apple pie. I've eaten three helpings of the stew and getting ready to eat another one. I felt a little better today – I'll probably have a good day tomorrow (Monday), since I have chemo on Tuesday. Gary doesn't think I'll be strong enough for chemo."

In the latter weeks of October, the breezes blew a brusque reality that the cancer was getting the upper hand as Dava was getting weaker and spending more time in bed during the daylight hours as well as night on a number of consecutive days. She was scheduled for a CT scan on October 28th, a Tuesday without chemo, and getting set up for a new type of chemo to begin on November 4th. The new chemo would have some possible side effects like numbness in the hands and feet, and gloves would be needed to protect the hands from anything cold. The doctor also said it was a little more toxic. That didn't sound like the kind of medicine for a weakened immune system, but what was the alternative?

It's Friday, October 31, 2008, Halloween, and Dava was not feeling well at all. Yesterday her mom and dad visited, and we got out of the house for a while. We came back home shortly because Dava just didn't feel well, and at bedtime she threw up. The early evening hours of that day are emblazoned in my brain. I was reading a book, and Dava was resting in her bed before the seven o'clock hour. Suddenly the sadness of the moment came upon me. I could still hear the trick or treaters down the street, and the lights were mostly out except for a lamp in the living room and the nightlights down the hallway. I put my book aside and picked up my journal in which I have written only on rare occasions, but on that night, I needed to write down my feelings:

"I feel very sad tonight because Dava has been feeling so bad. This week in which there was no chemo was supposed to be better. Last night as we were getting in bed around 9:30 she got sick to her stomach and threw up, don't know what brought that on, for Dava has eaten very little all week – It's Friday night & Halloween, she's in bed because she is just so

weak and I decided I want to make known that her not being in the living room with me at 7:00 o'clock is a very lonesome experience for me, so I know she must be extremely lonely plus the added tortures of pain going through her body. Pancreatic cancer has to rank as one of the very worse among any illness because it is absolutely relentless in its destruction of the body, and the mind has no recourse other than acceptance. Dava had a CT scan this past Tuesday, and we get the results on November 4th. We are both scared to ponder what it may show, for she has seemed so frail the past couple of weeks, though she looks beautiful as ever. The last few nights I have done some readings from Scripture and also from Portrait of a Lady *by Henry James, what an appropriate novel to be reading. How she has dealt with all the sickness and suffering these past thirteen months makes her the 'Ultimate Lady' in our household. – Hey, she just joined me in the living room for a piece of lemon pie."*

These moments were so special when Dava enjoyed a slight reprieve from the sickness, and so we sat together on the sofa, ate pie, and leaned on one another. I'm glad this journal entry of mine exists although I'll never be able to duplicate the feelings of *wanting* that appear in most of the text nor the exhilarating finish where I was surprised at her sudden appearance in the living room. But it makes the remembrances come alive for me, and the sadness turned to joy was as Keats may have discovered and expressed in his poem, "Welcome Joy, Welcome Sorrow." Here are just four lines:

Welcome joy, welcome sorrow
Lethe's weed and Hermes' feathers
Come to-day and come to- morrow
I do love you both together."

I'm venturing to say Lethe's weed and Hermes' feather is somewhere between deep despair and abundant hope. Regardless, they do come together, joy and sorrow, during the period of dealing with a terminal illness. It became clear to me that joy and sorrow are necessary to make one's life complete; it's not one or the other but both existing together.

On Saturday, November 1st, Dava noted in her journal:

"It's a beautiful day – if I could just get rid of the pain in my left back near my kidney – oh well, if that's all I've got to complain about. My CT scan results will be there Tuesday & I'm not exactly feeling good about that. If everything has stayed the same I'll be happy – I'm not able to eat or go to the bathroom & I have thrown up this past week a few times. I'm worried I'm going to turn into a chunk of petrified wood – I can't remember being so small."

This was the first scan that we were dreading to see the results; the one after her radiation in late July turned out to be an alarming amount of bad news concerning the

discovery of additional tumors; but, no, we were not necessarily thinking it was all going to be bad. Tuesday's doctor
visit was weighing on our minds because Dava was physically weakened and not getting much nourishment intake.

The journey beginning in November was like a roller
coaster ride into the abyss. Though Dava was far more frail
than during the summer months, she was still able to have
good days now and then, and it did not appear to me like
things would be coming apart at the seams as it soon did.
Her November 4th visit to the doctor was the first hurdle
of that month. Why do all the significant moments arrive
on the 4th of the month? I don't know, but they did, and it
continued to be the all-consuming date of the month, the
infamous fourth.

Dava and I left the house early on the fourth of November on our way to pick up my sister Mary Lee for our weekly
doctor visit. We were very weary and with some trepidation
concerning the test results and learning more about the
new chemo treatment. Once we had Mary Lee in the car,
she was able to distract our thoughts to other topics; after
all, how bad could the news be when compared to all the bad
news received over the past thirteen months? It started out
as a fairly routine office visit with blood tests and a short
waiting time before seeing Dr. Van Amburg. It's easy for me
to recreate the visual image that day in the examining room
which indicated that the news we were about to receive

would not be good at all, a situation unwillingly recalled time and again. Dr. Van Amburg was standing and examining Dava who was sitting up on the examining table, and I was on her left side. Debbie, the nurse practitioner, was also in the room which only happened rarely that both the doctor and nurse were there at the same time. My brother John and Mary Lee were standing behind us. Soon Dr. Van Amburg drew up a stool, and looking up at Dava, said that he had some troubling news. Her CT scan showed a blood clot. The sensation was almost like a bee sting, all eyes focused on Dava or the doctor with Dava immediately asking, "Could the blood clot go to my heart or brain?" Dr. Van Amburg said that the clot was in the vein leading to the liver from the pancreas and that it wouldn't attack the heart or the brain. We already knew the liver was damaged enough from the increasing number of tumors. The doctor then informed us that he would have Dava put on the blood thinner, Coumadin plus shots of Lovenox to try to keep the clot small and also prevent potential clots from forming.

Then Dava asked the doctor about the new type of chemo. He said the chemo would make her fingers numb, a type of neuropathy, that her hands would have to be protected against anything cold, to the point of wearing gloves while getting anything out of the refrigerator. Dava thought that sounded scary and said, "So the news is not too good at all." Dr. Van Amburg looked up at Dava from his stool and said, "You don't have to do any of this if you don't want to." And before Dava could answer, I responded, "Oh yes, we want to continue with the treatments." Dava just squeezed my hand. Dr. Van Amburg was being the gentle soul he could be at times, possibly realizing the status of her situation more clearly than either of us, but I just felt we were still in this fight and not wanting to yield, not yet anyway. I'm sure he did not want to put Dava through the rigors of a more toxic chemo session if she felt she had fought enough, and the blood clot was now another threat that had to be entered into the equation of whether to continue or not.

Dava's journal entry on Wednesday, November the 5th, referring to the doctor's visit:

"Went to see the doctor yesterday – not good news. There's a blood clot in the vein leading to the liver. Started me on a blood thinner – one is a shot to the stomach and other in pill form. Next Tuesday they start me on new chemo – only go once every three weeks & I will continue taking chemo pill. My liver enzymes are really high – over 700. We went by John's house after leaving doctor's for lunch – I threw up just as we were getting ready to eat. Threw up again last night at bedtime."

The news of the blood clot was quite devastating news to receive because Dava seemed to fear them the most throughout her treatments. So the blood thinning medicine Coumadin appeared to be the right course of action, or maybe the only way to manage the clot. I wasn't aware of all the risks with blood thinning medicine that I'm aware of now and became aware when it was beyond anyone's ability to control its destructive nature. Dava insisted on giving herself the shots to her stomach rather than relying on my abilities. Even with the practice I had of sticking the needle into the tennis ball as preparation, it was probably a wise decision on her part. Our grandchildren, Ethan and Emily, were visiting along with their mother Andrea as Dava gave herself the first shot in the stomach. Ethan who was three years old intently watched as his grandmother gave herself the shot saying, "Granny, I want to be a doctor now." Later that night when Dava took her Coumadin pill, she immediately became sick to her stomach and threw it up. Maybe that was an indication of something amiss or something we missed.

Dava was handling the shots and pills pretty well by the second night in that at least the pill stayed down. Now her worries turned toward the new chemo which would begin the next Tuesday. She noted in her journal on November 6th:

'I can only take new chemo once every three weeks, must be strong, it is to give me neuropathy in feet and hands, and

can't touch anything cold – I feel so sad for my Mom and Dad & my girls & Gary."

Dava and I traveled to the local hospital near us each morning for blood work since starting the Coumadin. On one occasion a student nurse, a young man, was assigned to draw Dava's blood. He was trying to get the blood drawn but was having no success, and I noticed Dava in tears. I simply said he would have to stop that Dava could not take the needle any longer. Dava assured the young man that she wasn't upset with him. She explained to him that she had been through so much. She shook the young nurse's hand, and the department manager apologized to us. The head nurse said that for very fragile patients, they always try to use very experienced nurses to draw blood and would the next time.

On Friday afternoon, my brother Rob called from Columbia, Missouri, saying he would be coming to De Soto on Saturday to stay with us, which was always nice to look forward to. Later that evening, my sister Judy called from California. She said that she and Mark had thought about flying in to visit us on her birthday, December 13th. I'm not sure if I stammered a bit or what, but Judy just as quickly added, "Or do you think we ought to come sooner?" Dava was resting on the sofa, and I said something like yes, I think that would be better. Judy was so sweet, without any further questions she said that they would come next week, and I said, "You want to tell Dava?" Dava wrote in her journal that Friday night: *"Judy called, said she and Mark are flying in to visit me, they are so good to use their time and money to come see me."*

It's difficult for me to read Dava's November 8th entry in her journal, for it is the last entry in her home journals. She did write a few more times in a smaller journal in the hospital, but this was her last one at home:

"Have laid around most of the day, while Gary has done laundry, dishes, and the bathrooms. Mary Lee fixed grilled cheese & sliced me a pear – so good. – Rob is coming tonight – I don't seem to even have enough strength to take a shower anymore – Gary has been helping me as best he can. He puts lotion on my legs & back. Not many husbands could put up with my s—t."

Actually, I was doing what spouses have been doing for ages, helping the one they love most in this world get through a rough period. As for as the journal entry itself, I always find myself flipping through the few unused pages to see if I might discover a later note or notations, and I'm still doing that, but that was the final one.

It appeared that everything was going well on Saturday as Dava continued her shots and later on would take her pill of Coumadin. Rob arrived later in the afternoon, and I fixed a spaghetti meal while he and Dava solved some word puzzles together, something they both enjoyed doing and were really good at it. It was nearly eleven o'clock that night before we started heading to our bedrooms. Rob had just said good night and closed the door to the bedroom, and Dava and I were getting ready for bed when she said, "Get the bucket!" and I held it while she spit up a silver dollar size spittle of blood into the bucket. She was very scared and made a point of telling me it didn't come from her throat but that she threw this up from her stomach. I went to Rob's room and told him Dava had spit up blood and that I was getting ready to call the doctor to see what we should do.

This was that scenario that I began near the beginning of this book. It was almost like the beginning of the end, but we neither one was thinking that. We were just really upset with what was happening. How could such a good day's adventure in happiness turn on a dime and leave us in an abyss? By coincidence, the doctor on night calls that week-end was Dava's doctor, Dr. Van Amburg. When I related that Dava had thrown up a spittle of blood from her stomach, he said, "Oh shit, take her to the emergency room and take no more Coumadin."

It didn't take the three of us long to get on our way to St. Luke's Hospital emergency room. I'm glad Rob was with us at this late hour. It sort of spread the concern to three from just us two. Rob's presence and support was a calming effect on our fifty minute ride to the hospital. The emergency room staff examined Dava as she was telling them what had occurred and about her regimen of Coumadin she was taking. I'm not quite sure what tests were performed that night, but we were there about an hour and a half before Dava was released to go home.

I was not aware at the time of the deadly, potential effects of blood thinners and what they could do to a damaged and weakened system that Dava was living with at that stage. It wasn't a large amount of blood loss, but Dava made sure that I and the doctors knew it came from her stomach. We arrived home after two in the morning and knew that we all needed some sleep, but by morning we discovered that none of us could manage to get the kind of sleep desired. There were too many thoughts twisting and turning in our heads for that. What did this new development of spitting up blood mean? Was it a one-time occurrence? What would the doctors come up with next?

chapter seventeen

The Final Weeks and Days

On the Sunday and Monday following the emergency room visit, our world got back to what was considered normal after the diagnosis thirteen months ago. The spitting up blood episode did not register with me as being possibly the catastrophic event that it was, and it didn't register with Dava either although it scared her a lot at the time. With no chemo this past week, Dava had these couple of her so-called good days but was now having to fret about receiving the new, more toxic chemo on the next Tuesday. And even though she was more frail than she had been in those previous months, Dava's ability to enjoy her good days was still there, and her determination to take whatever came her way was still there.

Tuesday, November 11th arrived, and Dava and I picked up my sister Mary Lee and headed to St. Luke's for Dava's weekly doctor's visit with the new chemo on the agenda. There was not much conversation about the Saturday night blood spit-up, other than the fact that there were no more incidences after she stopped taking the Coumadin. The emphasis now dealt with preparing for this new chemo treatment. So it was off to start the first of this more toxic chemo dripped into Dava's system. The room was exactly the same with the same number of patients and nurses as usual, but the one big difference was in the bag hanging overhead, and we didn't know how different the results on Dava's system would be. The chemo session lasted about the same amount of time as before, and soon we were headed straight home because Dava said she was really tired.

It wasn't long after we started our journey home that Mary Lee and I noticed a different effect this treatment was having on Dava's overall composure. She could hardly hold her head up, so Mary Lee who was seated in the backseat braced her hands behind the back of Dava's head so as to steady her. She became more and more agitated and restless as we got closer to De Soto. Mary Lee was still holding Dava's head to help her relax as we approached my sister's house. Mary Lee suggested we just continue on to my house and that she could drive back after Dava got settled at home, but I assured her that we only had the five-mile trip, and I thought that we could make it alright. After leaving her house and driving to Highway E, a hilly road with a lot of huge curves, Dava began saying, "Let me out of here," and reaching for the door handle. I leaned her toward me and began telling her to hang on for five more minutes and that we were near our home in Summer Set. She was absolutely miserable. She flailed her arms and again repeated, "Get me out of here," and I just kept a tight grip on her left arm and kept assuring her that we would be home very soon.

After arriving home, Dava was totally exhausted and yet very restless. I held her up as she draped her arms around my neck, totally leaning on me. We slowly inched our way back to our bedroom. I laid her on the bed, and she was out. The restlessness had left her, and she was sleeping as I positioned the covers over her. I left her in the clothes she had on, just removing her coat and shoes. She was resting which was what she really needed, so I kissed her lips and let her sleep. I then called Mary Lee to let her know what had happened and that I should have listened to her about getting Dava settled first before dropping her off. Dava had never been this way with the other chemo treatments right after receiving the dosage. There were days after receiving the other chemo where she was totally weakened to the point of not being able to raise herself off the sofa, but that was the second or third day after the treatment. She was in a state of delirium during that ride home and until she lay on the bed to rest.

It was a beautiful fall Wednesday, November 12, 2008,

and I fixed Dava an egg on buttered toast to serve her while she sat up in bed, and she managed to eat all of it. She dressed, and we lingered in the living room for a while. I vacuumed the carpets and did a load of laundry. For the most part, we were content to just sit together and feel a sense of relief that the day had started off so well. Dava was feeling fairly good despite the new chemo effects of yesterday. Just after eleven o'clock, Mary Lee called asking how Dava was doing. I informed her that Dava was having a really good day so far and had eaten all of her breakfast, and other than the normal back pain, she was feeling quite good. Mary Lee was pleased with the news and said she was fixing something that I could pick up later in the day. So everything seemed to be in working harmony. One of these kinds of days one treasures, especially when there are so many disorderly ones to even things out.

One minute all is bliss, and soon our world is amiss. For it was no more than fifteen minutes after I hung up from talking to my sister that the lovely lightness of the day suddenly turned toward the darkness of night. Everything seemed so perfect, too perfect I guess, considering Dava's condition. She was half-way energetic, smiling, and wanting to help with the laundry. I emptied the dryer's contents into two tubs and was carrying them back to the bedroom. The next several minutes proved to be Dava's last minutes together with me at our home. As I entered our bedroom, I set the tubs of laundry on the bed, and before I could completely turn toward Dava, she hollered out, *"Get my bucket!"* I ran to the living room and snatched her bucket as she sat on the edge of the bed. I held the bucket for her as she vomited. But what came forth was not undigested food but pure blood that filled the whole bottom of the gray, plastic bucket. The whole scene was beyond anything I could ever imagine; it was surreal. I can't express the anguish in my heart that the love of my life was having to go through such a horrific experience. It is not enough to say we were scared; we were terrified. Dava then asked me to get a baggy and a spoon, so she could preserve the clots for the doctor to see. They were the size of egg yolks. I said to Dava that we needed to head for the hospital, and Dava asked me to call Mary Lee.

First, I called one of the girls and told her what had happened and that we were heading to St Luke's. I called Mary Lee about the incident but did not request her going since two of our daughters were riding with us, and Carrie was following us in her car. The drive to the hospital was a harrowing experience. I realized the urgency to get my wife to the hospital, and maybe I should have called an ambulance, but I thought I could have her there in about the same amount of time. I was speeding 70 to 80 miles per hour on the interstate and being careful and cautious as we raced to our goal, the hospital. After we turned onto Highway 141, the traffic became heavier, even at the noon hour. We were stopped at a red light when Dava asked for the bucket again. This time it was pure blood, not clots. She just filled the bottom of the bucket with pure red blood. Dava looked up at me and said in a weak voice, "Get me to the hospital." She knew she had lost a lot of blood and was scared; we all were. As the light changed to green, the girls suggested I put on my flashers which I did, and I also moved to the far left passing lane. A couple of cars moved over out of our way; however, one car stayed in our lane moving at a moderate speed. With my flashers flashing and moving closer to his rear bumper, I lightly tapped my horn. Still, the driver would not go over to the other lane even though he had room. With my three girls in the car witnessing their mother regurgitating blood, this guy from his car looks over at us giving us the middle finger as we passed him. My first thought was that he had no idea what we are dealing with in this emergency, and neither my daughters nor I have forgotten the gesture he gave us that day. It reminds one of man's inhumanity to man, but my mission was to get Dava to the hospital as quickly as I could, so I ignored him.

Fifteen minutes later, I was pulling into the emergency room lot at St Luke's Hospital. The girls got out with their mom while I parked the car. I met my brother John and sister-in-law Onie waiting inside the emergency room door. They had seen the blood in the bucket as the girls helped their mother to a cubicle. By the time I entered the room, Dava was already hooked up to fluids and was getting prepared for a blood transfusion. She was surrounded in her bed by a number of doctors, and one of the nurses told me that Dava was below eight pints which requires a blood transfusion. I was just relieved that there was not a third incident of throwing up blood and that the medical people would see that she was stabilized. After the transfusion was completed, Dava was admitted to the Intensive Care Unit, and I remained in the waiting room until I could get in to see her. There were about seven or eight of my family there in the waiting room with me and the girls. I recall my brother John asking, "Gary, don't you think Dava's had enough chemo and maybe she can't handle anymore?" I informed him that the chemo was not the cause at all but that the internal bleeding was the effect of the Coumadin blood thinner she had been taking for the blood clot. I added that the bleeding and loss of blood is the main problem now, and I don't know yet what the doctors can do to stop it.

After Dava was settled in the ICU, I was able to go in and visit with her. She was very alert and appeared replenished and having a nurse at her station at all times made her feel safe and comfortable there. We were still trying to ascertain what this all meant and discussing how suddenly our day had changed at the eleven o'clock hour. It was now about

2:30 p.m. Two people were allowed to visit in the ICU at one time, so the girls, Mary Lee, or I were always back there with Dava until 7:00 p.m. after which no visitors were allowed in the ICU.

It was to be a very long and restless night for me. I found an empty loveseat in one of the corners of the waiting room near the entrance in the event that someone needed to contact me. Around nine o'clock I curled up on it thinking sleep. I noticed that there was another family group in the waiting room who were very talkative, and the lights were still up bright. I lay there trying to get some sleep amid the thoughts of the day, the other family's loud talking, and the bright lights. Around eleven o'clock the lights dimmed, and the room was a lot quieter, but when I had almost fallen asleep, a member of the other family started the talking again, and the lights brightened. It was another hour before the lights dimmed, and it was quiet enough for me to eventually drop off into sleep. I awoke several more times that night which brings to mind the words from Simon and Garfunkel's "Bridge Over Troubled Waters." For I suspect all the reasons expressed in that song, feeling sorry for my Dava who had suffered so much that day and feeling sorry for myself and the girls because we felt we were in the midst of troubled waters, made my restless night worse. So it was near four o'clock in the morning before I really drifted off into a deep sleep, only to be awakened by unwelcome news.

About six o'clock in the morning, Dr. Cort was waking me in a soft tone, saying, "Mr. Doyen, I need to talk to you." The room was eerily quiet and very dark, just night lights, and the doctor whispered as I awoke. I sat up quickly, stunned somewhat at the thought of what he had to tell me so urgently at such an early hour. I knew Dr. Cort only because he performed my colonoscopy earlier in August of this year. He began by telling me that the cancer was nearing the aorta and that Dr. Van Amburg had done a good job of keeping the cancer from overtaking Dava, but now there was the bleeding, and he didn't know if it could be stopped and that we could be getting near the end. He continued by saying he would proceed with an endoscopy around eight o'clock this morning but wanted me to know he wasn't sure what he would find, nor was he sure he would be able to stop the bleeding from her stomach that was like a giant ulcer. I recall telling him I hoped he would be able to stop Dava's bleeding, to which he replied that he would do everything possible. After he left, I was sitting alone on the loveseat, alone with the quietness, the darkness, and fear of the unknown. For the first time that feeling of *alone* was all over me. I was alone, and the person I loved the most was in a very precarious situation and at the mercy of the doctors and the Good Lord. We both were.

I wanted so badly to get back into the ICU to see Dava but was told that she was being taken to the outpatient area for the endoscopy and that I could see her before she went in for the procedure. I was still reeling a bit from the early morning visit from Dr. Cort and felt I needed to share the news with the girls. Three of my daughters were teachers, and Andrea was helping me out at the furniture and appliance store, and I told them I would keep them all updated throughout the morning, and if I thought they needed to leave their jobs for any reason, I would let them know. It was nearing seven-thirty that morning when the staff rolled Dava down the hallway where I was waiting for her to enter the preparation area. It had been thirteen hours since we saw each other, but with the added knowledge received this morning, it seemed like a weekend if not a whole week since we kissed and touched one another. Dava said the good night's sleep was what she needed, and knowing the nurse was watching over her all night gave her comfort.

The endoscopy procedure lasted about an hour total, and a male nurse was the first to approach me and said he thought everything went well and that Dr. Cort sealed up some bleeding areas. Soon Dr. Cort appeared and said that all went well, and he had sealed off two areas where there was bleeding. He continued by saying that he might have to do the procedure again if any areas were missed. It was going to take a few days to see if Dava's blood loss diminished; however, my overall feeling after the endoscopy was somewhat more hopeful than earlier that morning. I called Andrea and informed her that the doctor seemed pleased that the procedure went so well. By now I was alongside Dava in the recovery area where she was just coming to from the anesthesia. I kissed her and told her that the doctor was quite confident that he got the areas of the bleeding sealed. We held each other's hands and were just happy to be together. The nurse came to take her back to ICU where I was able to stay with her for most of the day. My brother Mick and sister-in-law Peggy visited us that day. There was no need for a blood transfusion on Thursday, so it appeared that her stomach was successfully sealed.

On Friday afternoon November 14th, Mark and Judy arrived from California and came straight to the hospital with Mary Lee. Both had good visits with Dava in the ICU and later that early evening suggested I go home and get a good night's rest. Mark drove my vehicle, and he, Judy, and I traveled to my house, but first Mark stopped by his favorite St. Louis store, Dierbergs, and bought what seemed like a week's supply of groceries. I certainly wasn't going to go hungry on his watch. It was so great having them in during this critical time. They got me home and situated and said they would be out early next morning to head back to the hospital to see Dava.

It was around eight thirty in the evening, and I was

sitting on a stool at the kitchen bar snacking on some of the delicacies Mark had purchased when it dawned on me that I should update some very good friends in Paducah, Kentucky. Two of my best friends from there were Connie and Sam Leone. Connie and I sang quite often together in our church choir, but I had not seen her since April 2007.

Dava and I had stopped by for a visit on our return from a business trip. It had been fifteen years since we left Paducah, and we had not really kept in touch except for that visit. When Dava was first diagnosed with the cancer, I placed a call to our previous parish church and told the then secretary, a member of our singing group, the news about Dava and requested her to tell the others. But this night I placed the call to Sam and Connie and received a voice mail. I began explaining that Dava had taken a turn for the worse this week and was in ICU, and before I could say another word, Connie picked up the phone and said, "Oh no, Gary, what happened to Dava?" She was near crying by the sound of her voice. I told her that Dava has been dealing with pancreatic cancer for thirteen months. Connie was crying as she talked, saying, "I didn't know anything about Dava being sick." I then said that I had informed the secretary and told her to tell everyone. After briefly filling her in on the latest circumstances of Dava's throwing up the blood, I too was sobbing and so choked up I could barely get through the next sentence. Connie just kept saying, "I'm so sorry, I'm so sorry." I could feel her anguish, sorrow, and compassion with every word she spoke. She said she would let the others know of Dava's situation, and they would all pray for us. I thanked her and hung up the phone with both of us sobbing while saying our goodbyes. It was an especially difficult call because I thought she already knew of Dava's serious illness. I recall the last time we visited Connie in April 2007, when the three of us had lunch, and I took a picture of Dava and Connie together. When Connie answered the phone, her voice communicated both surprise and grief and made me realize that soon I will lose my darling Dava which brought sobs and tears to me as well. I was grateful for her sincerity and compassion toward me, and even though it was a sad phone call, my heart swelled just knowing that another was taking it as I, myself, was taking it.

I'm presently writing during the month of November, the same time frame as the happenings some ten years ago. The effect on my senses—the shades of cloudiness and early darkness, the smells—garners up the heightened emotions that this particular time of year can generate and is of immense importance. The many recent cold damp days, though Dava loved them, would have chilled her to the bone during her illness. I light a candle like she often did during this month. The scent takes me back in time, and the setting of the clocks back tonight reminds me of Dava's desiring the morning light instead of light fading into early darkness. And lastly, our knowing that this late autumn will lead us into winter when life is stilled and dormant.

Dava remained in ICU for three more days where she continued to receive blood transfusions about every third day or when it was required. On the 18th of November she was moved to the seventh floor, the cancer floor at St. Luke's, to room 7707. This move allowed me to be with her around the clock which I liked very much, and Dava was happy being together too, although she said the ICU did comfort her because of the close and continual attention it provided. For the most part, Dava was eating fairly well. The morphine was keeping the pain at bay, but she had blood in her bowel movements. She once had me check her bowel movement, and there was dark, red blood present. The loss of blood was our most immediate and deepest concern. When we asked Dr. Van Amburg if this was residue remaining in her stomach or was it new blood, he simply said he was not sure but that he and his staff were monitoring that. Dava's journal entry in her hospital journal on November 19th reads:

> "Didn't sleep as well on the 7th floor as I did in ICU, I knew I had someone watching me at all times practically. The two male nurses I had last night were pretty good, Oh and the workers on this floor remember Gary, who doesn't? And Gary was invited to stay at John and Onie's last night – he went for

dinner but he told John he wanted to go back to the hospital to be with me, so he came back to the hospital soon after dinner – My blood count today was 7.9, so Dr. Cleary ordered a new pint of blood & I have a new morphine patch put on today too! John has been here most of the morning – he gives Gary good company."

On Thursday morning, Dr. Van Amburg was making his rounds and checking on Dava around seven-thirty; and soon Dr. Phillips, Dava's longtime primary physician, also came into the room. Both were chatting with one another off to the side of the room and then mentioned to me that they might consider another endoscopy but would first check with Dr. Cleary who was in Dr. Cort's office. When Dava recognized that the doctors were talking quietly to me, she began thinking something was wrong. For no sooner had both doctors left and I went to sit on the edge of her bed, she said, "I'm dying, aren't I." I told her that no one has ever said that to me, and if they did, I would tell her if she asked. I said that they were considering another endoscopy but were not sure until they checked with Dr. Cleary. To hear her say those words just made me cringe; it was very sad and heart wrenching to hear the one I love most of all talk of dying. I was not prepared to let go at this point, and she accepted the truth when I told her, but she knew more about how she felt, and maybe that led to her question.

Dava's overall condition was in fact getting worse day by day. During the night of November 21st, Dava kept asking me for water about every twenty minutes. Then I would watch her drift off to sleep as I reclined on my cot. After another twenty minutes or so, she would say, "I'm thirsty." On November 22nd, Dava asked me to look at how much her legs had swollen. It appeared that the fluids were building up inside her. I began to think that these last few days were a turning point that Dava could not reverse. Her system may have started shutting down certain organs. She now had to be bathed in bed, and she was sleeping a lot more than before.

Early the following week, Monday or Tuesday, Dr. Van Amburg was making his rounds and checking Dava while reviewing her blood work. When he had finished and Dava had just received some morphine and was sleeping, he asked me to step out into the corridor. He said that he did not think I would want Dava on a respirator if it came to that point because of her advanced cancer. I answered, "No, I wouldn't want her on a respirator." He then said he would have to note that in Dava's records at the main nurse's station. He spoke in his regular soft tone, and I answered in a whispered voice because I knew how acute Dava's hearing was, and I was concerned she might hear our conversation. When I reentered the room, she was sleeping soundly. Even though that may be a routine question that doctors are required to ask about one's loved one, it is a lot different when it's the actual love one who hears it. I felt really sad at that moment, looking at Dava and touching her face with my fingers. Although the doctor didn't say anything like she was dying, just that if it suddenly turned that way, no respirator would be used. In other words, she would be leaving us.

Here we were just a couple of days before Thanksgiving, so I asked Dr. Van Amburg if there was any chance I could get Dava home for that day. He replied, "Being home isn't always what it is cracked up to be, and Dava needs what the hospital can give her, and your insurance people are agreeable with her being here." Though I accepted his opinion, I asked Dava what she thought of spending the holiday at home, and she said that she would prefer to stay at the hospital. My desire was for her to see our home again, to lie in her bed, and have the girls and grandkids near her. All those wishes were running through my mind. It is heartbreaking for me to think of that Wednesday when we headed to the hospital, unaware that Dava would never return to our home again. I truly believed that Dava would have loved to see our home again, but her condition made it nearly impossible.

Thanksgiving week was upon us. This was always that time of year when Dava excelled in making the holiday celebrations the memorable days they were. She made every Thanksgiving and Christmas a delightful time to look forward to with all her decorating, along with the season's varied scents that were abundantly distributed throughout our home. Every holiday celebration for these many years had taken place at our home with our daughters, grandchildren, and some extended family present. Our home was the place to be at this time of year, and I loved it.

Thinking back, I recall one Thanksgiving that remains especially memorable for me. It was our first since moving back to De Soto in early 1993 and moving into a newly built house in Liberty Ridge subdivision, just a mile or so north of town. Early that morning, Dava was up, and the aroma of turkey and dressing along with the spices were already filling the air. My thoughts drift back to that day. How festive it all was with the kids and grandkids and the smell of turkey, cranberries, and pumpkin pies! But most important was the spirit of love and togetherness that was so infectious. It wasn't long before two of my brothers, Pat and Rob, stopped by to say hello. They had come to town to enjoy a Thanksgiving dinner at our sister Mary Lee's house but decided to stop by our place earlier that morning. Pat had brought a treasure of vinyl records of opera recordings, and soon the whole house was being serenaded by Pavarotti and others while Dava busied herself in the kitchen. Now and then she would show up with a bite of this or a sip of that, and as we shared in the sounds of the operatic voices,

Dava concentrated on her preparations. I remember all my Thanksgiving Day celebrations because they all had one unique beginning, Dava. She was the light that ushered in the day for the rest of our family; she was the spark that lit up our world, especially at this time of year. When I think too much about those holidays with Dava, my thoughts turn to tears, tears of joy and gratitude.

For most of Thursday, November 27th, it was a regular day in the hospital room. Our girls planned a late afternoon Thanksgiving dinner for us in room 7707. Dava had hardly eaten anything the past couple of days, and the day started out very lackluster. But after our daughters completed Thanksgiving dinner with their immediate families, they arrived in full force with an abundance of turkey, dressing, potatoes and gravy, and all kinds of pies like pumpkin and pecan included in the selection. Their mother had been resting and sleeping most of the day. Her condition made her much weaker with no appetite, but in no time, the girls had their mom sitting up in bed and filling her a plate with all the fixings; she proceeded to start eating. I'm not sure if it was for their sake that she consumed a fair portion of the food on her plate, but I do know she had not eaten well at all the previous few days. There were some photos taken that day, and Dava looked as though she was enjoying her dinner. I also know that she was giving the performance of her life to not disappoint anyone. That was just Mom's way.

Sarah, my youngest daughter, made me a framed collage of photos from Thanksgiving Day and through the weekend. There are poses of her with her mom, me with mom, and the grandkids with their grandmother; even though Dava's frailty and weakness are evident, her loveliness and strength of will come right out at you as you stare at the pictures. I hung that collage on the wall directly in front of my treadmill. When I think that I can't do another two minutes, I glance up at that framed collage, and I'm not only able to continue on but to get revved up, for I know that the pain I feel is temporary and quite insignificant compared to what Dava endured daily from sunrise to sunset. Just like when she was with me, she remains my source for strength and endurance. The day Sarah gave me the framed collage of her mom that weekend, I hesitated as to where I would hang it, for it showed Dava in a very weakened state. I didn't want that image of her to be viewed by others on the mantle or the living room wall, so I found this special place above the treadmill to provide me each morning with the love, strength, and remembrances of our last Thanksgiving together.

The girls took turns staying with their mother and me over the Thanksgiving weekend, so when she needed help to sit up or be given water during the night, we were all there to comfort her. They were spoiling their mom with massages, including her head and face. Dava's hairdresser,

Mona, came to the hospital on Sunday the 30th to cut and style her thin, graying curls. She even managed to cut mine; when I offered her money, she refused. I told her that it was a tip, not a payment, but she still refused by saying that she wanted to do this for Dava and me. Mona is such a sweet person. She made it fun for all of us the minute she showed up, and I couldn't thank her enough.

The daughters and grandkids were with Dava nearly all day Sunday, and even though she was very tired, she relished holding the little ones' hands and having them near her. It wasn't anything like our past Thanksgiving celebrations with Dava taking the lead, but she was at the very center of this special, memorable Thanksgiving. She used the little energy she had to touch a hand, give a little kiss, or with the raising of a finger, point out the passing of an angel.

On Sunday evening of the last day of November, Dava and I were again alone, just the two of us. Each day she was losing the strength to do much more than sit up for a few minutes, only to recline soon after to sleep which was induced by the morphine drip. That night Dava asked me to read to her from Scripture, and I began reading from one book to another, just fragments from Psalms, Ecclesiastes and Wisdom. Then I recalled that Dava at times during her journey had this yearning and hope that Jesus would find her worthy enough to accept her into His home. And as I sat by her bed with her fading in and out of sleep, I asked God to help me find a passage from the Word that would comfort her. I then opened the Bible to read from John's First Letter, Chapter 4, and the words, staring me in the eyes was this title, "God's Love and Ours." It reads as follows:

> "Beloved, let us love one another because love is of God.
> Everyone who loves is begotten of God and has knowledge of God.
> The man without love has known nothing of God, for God is love.
> God's love was revealed in our midst in this way:
> He sent His only Son to the world that we may have life through Him.
> Love, then, consists in this: not that we have loved God,
> but that He has loved us. Love has no room for fear,
> rather perfect love casts out all fear, and since fear has to do with punishment, love is not yet perfect in one who is afraid."

After reading the passage from John's First Epistle, I said to Dava that I had found the words she needed to hear. She listened to these reassuring words, and then I reinforced the reading by saying, "It wasn't your being worthy enough, but more importantly His love for you was enough, for you have given love beyond measure to the lengths of your outstretched arms just as He did." She just looked at me and smiled and then slipped off to sleep. It is such moments as this one that keep my faith above water. I needed help at that moment to help Dava, and it was given to me. I may have read that passage before at home or at Mass, but that night it opened itself to me when I asked for it in my desire to comfort my love.

Andrea's journal entry on November 30th, 2008:

"Haven't written in over three months, a lot has happened w/Mom. She's been in the hospital almost three weeks now – we brought her up on a Wednesday. She was throwing up blood, bad. The emergency room took her right in. She was in ICU for 1 and ½ weeks – now she's in room 7707 since and only getting worse. She has swelling due to gaining fluids, and her stomach leaks blood. I've been to see her everyday – she is so weak – she can't even get up to pee she hurts so bad. Dad told me and Carrie that they want to bring her home. She asked about going home on Tuesday of this week for some reason. Hospice would come and be there to keep her comfortable "as they say." Do they think it would be better for her to be home to die? Dad explained that once home, she can't receive blood anymore, and they wouldn't draw off the fluids. She would eventually, within a day likely either have an extreme blood loss and will die or drown in her own fluids and her heart will go into cardiac arrest. The doctors asked if dad and us girls could handle the throwing up of blood and her

death at home. Dad said we could and would. We will put her in a hospital bed and someone would be with her around the clock. It's so selfish of me, but I don't want to do this – I don't want her to die – I know the hospital can't keep her forever. She's in pain, she's scared to die and I think scared to go home – I've lost close friends in the past, but I have never hurt like this, my family, my Mom is my life. – I'm not sure that everyone gets us – "our family" – We are all very close – very close! She doesn't deserve this, nor does Dad – watch over both of them. No one could ask for a better Mom – I hope she knows the love I have for her. I will miss her dearly."

chapter eighteen

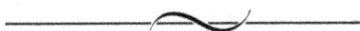

Dava Lets Go

The month of December was now upon us, and it had always been one of the favorite months of the year for Dava and me. How ironic is it that December delivered the fatal decree in Dava's journey? Maybe it was predestined to be, that we should be separated from one another at a time when we were oneness in spirit with all the feelings that are deepened in December. For every emotion, whether sentimental or through the purity of our love, was expressed during the holiday season, especially in December. As the first of its days arrived, the situation was no different than the past three weeks with the exception that Dava became increasingly weaker. The girls made the trip from De Soto around five o'clock after their workday, and the atmosphere in the hospital room was enlivened by their being there. They gathered around their mother and could not get enough of her presence, nor could Dava get enough of them. I sat back in a chair just watching as they hovered over her and listened to every word she spoke to them.

It was sometime beyond the time of their arrival, and all were standing near Mom's bedside doing various activities to make her more comfortable when Dava called out to them to gather around her. I'm not sure she called my name, but she wanted us to gather around her bed. She wanted to say something. I stayed back as she talked to the girls. I later asked our daughters what their mom had said exactly that night. Sarah told me that her mom had asked them if they thought she should keep fighting this thing or was it okay if she gave up the fight, for she was so weak. They all began answering her by saying that they wanted her to do whatever she felt she needed to do. Then their mother said she loved them so much and that it was so hard to let go, but maybe the time had come to let go. I had not heard the words spoken in her weakened breath, but I wanted her to live as long as she could; but she was more aware of her condition than we were. The girls stayed until the nine o'clock visiting hour had ended. When I look back on it, it was a memorable and special night for Dava, the girls, and me.

All night Monday Dava was asking for water every fifteen minutes, and when I would put the straw to her lips, she did not have enough strength to take the water up through the straw. It would go about three-fourths the way up, then only halfway, and soon she was out of breath. All I could think about was reflecting on the story of Jesus on the cross before he died and gave up His spirit and said, "I thirst." That thought entered my spirit, and I wondered if this was when Dava was beginning her final struggle or was it just like the last several nights when she asked me for water. When I mentioned to her that she wasn't getting the water to her mouth, she kept trying but only getting a weaker sip each time. I used a washcloth full of ice pressed against her lips, so she could suck the moisture from it. I continued this method of providing water for her most of the night.

Around six o'clock on Tuesday, December 2nd, I was awakened in a startling fashion by Dava who was sitting up and hollering, "Get me out of here!" I hurried over to ask her what she wanted, and she repeated, "Get me out of here." I asked her if she meant she wanted out of her bed or out of the hospital. As I looked into her eyes, she spoke as if she were in a stupor; again she said, "Get me out of here," not looking at me in the eyes but looking past me. I pushed the nurse's button as I turned her sideways with her legs hanging off the side of the bed where I held her in my arms. I then said to her, "Honey, you don't have the strength to get out of bed, just hold on to me." After she settled down a little, I laid her back on her pillow. Two male nurses arrived, and I informed them that she seemed to have difficulty breathing and was needing to sit up. One of the nurses said that her oxygen level was fine, and I added that maybe the air was not getting to her lungs, for she was struggling and not comfortable. Her on duty nurse soon came to the room and checked Dava and informed me that she was due more morphine which would make her more comfortable. Dava was now lying there seemingly at rest, so apparently the morphine did ease her difficulty breathing. I stood by her bedside watching her breathe in and out and looking so peaceful once the morphine took effect. But I will never forget the stare she gave me when I asked her what was wrong. She looked past me toward the wall and spoke, but her eyes never connected with mine. It was so mysterious and sad because she looked right through me and not at me.

It wasn't long after the nurse's departure that Dr. Van Amburg came into the room on his seven o'clock rounds. The tall lanky figure with the wavy, gray hair approached my cot where I was sitting and sat down beside me. The words he spoke were not what I was expecting to hear. In a very serious and demonstrative tone, "You need to know she may not make it through the day." I quickly replied, "Oh no, are you sure?" He then explained that Dava had weakened considerably of late, and he didn't think she could survive the day. No matter what was said, I was just not wanting to accept the finality of his words. I then said to him, "I'm not ready for that," but his voice was silent, and I realized that the end of everything in this fight against the cancer was at hand. Dava was lying peacefully under the influence of the morphine as the doctor left the room. He had taken a few minutes of his precious time to talk with me and tell me what needed to be told, and I knew that he had done all he could do for Dava. Although the news was difficult to bear, I was thankful for all his efforts and compassion at such a tragic time in my life.

It was imperative of me at this point to call our daughters and pass on the inevitable news the doctor had just related to me. I did call them and delivered the tragic news that the doctor doubted their mother would survive the day. Soon after, I phoned her parents concerning the doctor's prognosis. They had planned on coming to the hospital Monday, but the weather had turned bad, so they decided to wait until today. It was ironic and sad since Dava was still conscious on Monday had they been able to make it up on that day. Within a couple of hours, the girls with the grandkids were in our room. Her parents arrived a little later with Dava's aunt and uncle. Some of my brothers and Mary Lee were also present. The room was full.

On that Tuesday December 2nd, many of the family were gathered around Dava's bed, and I was standing at the head of the bed and hoping to hear her speak. She was sleeping so silently but suddenly spoke out, "Is my Mom and Dad here?" I let her know that they were sitting right behind me near her bed. I had them stand, and they placed their hands within Dava's hands. Sarah felt bad because she was kneeling in bed with her mom and somehow managed to kneel on Dava's leg. Dava said, "Get off me," and Sarah later said she wished that had not been the last words her mother spoke to her. About one-thirty in the afternoon, my niece, Erica, bent down close to her Aunt Dava's face telling her, "I have to go feed my baby, but I wanted to say I love you." I heard Dava reply, *"And I love you too."* Those were the last words I heard Dava speak, and last words are important to recognize. Her words, "And I love you too," are as good as any can ever be, for love is the gift that rises above all others; Dava gave her love to the very end of her life.

So there were nearly thirty of us in the room that Tuesday watching over Dava as she lay near death. I was hoping to hear her speak or open her eyes, but she was not able to do either. As late evening arrived, I suggested to her mother and father and aunt and uncle that if they needed to leave for home and get some rest, I would keep them posted on Dava's condition. They decided to leave around eight o'clock, but most of the families stayed until ten o'clock. It was about this time that I asked one of the nurses what we might expect. She said she didn't believe anything would happen soon, that Dava's heartbeat was strong. So with that news, everyone except the girls and me soon headed for home. The girls took turns lying next to their mother in her bed; at times, I took my turn lying close to her. As I looked at her, she was still so beautiful. I listened and watched her whispered breathing slide through her lips while gently rubbing my fingers across her face. I wanted to lie as close to her as I could and hoped that she could feel my presence without my causing her any discomfort. I wasn't sure she could know that I was there beside her, for she was so silently sleeping.

Later that night one of the nurses came to the room to check on Dava, and I asked her if there was any chance that Dava would regain consciousness. The nurse then asked me to follow her to the nurse's station where she showed me Dava's last blood test results. She pointed out that the measurement for albumin serum is supposed to be at 4.0 and anything below 3.0 is critical. Dava's was 2.4. That meant her liver was not functioning properly, and her whole system was slowly shutting down. I still didn't want to accept that the end was near, but now I realized it was soon to be.

Andrea's journal entry for December 3rd, 2008, reads as follows:

"Fourteen months tomorrow since we found out Mom has cancer – she's still in the hospital, three weeks today. Sarah called me Tuesday morning, yesterday, around 8:45 and said to get to the hospital that Mom has less than 24 hours to live.

Here we are, over 48 hours and she's still here. She looked so pitiful when we got here, her mouth open, eyes half-opened – she had no idea we were there (though they claim she can hear us). She came up from her bed a few times thru the night in a distant stare, yelling that she wanted out, trying to climb out of bed. They loaded her up w/ morphine – to a level 4."

In the early morning of December 3rd, the girls were bathing their mom and putting lotion on her body where they could see blue and purple areas developing. Dava was still breathing quite well when Dr. Phillips, her heart doctor, came to check on her. He proclaimed, "There certainly isn't anything wrong with her heart." That statement was so very true in so many ways. It wasn't long before Room 7707 was again filled with mostly my family watching over Dava as she silently slept. All of us knew she was still with us, for her breathing kept up at a strong and steady pace.

Later that evening after most of those visiting had left, Kay Beiser, my first cousin and a registered nurse associated with another hospital, came by to visit Dava, the girls, and me. As soon as she greeted us, she went directly to Dava and held her hand. She spoke to her as though Dava was hearing every word; as Kay later told us, she may very well have heard what she said. Kay was telling us that her hearing would be there right up to the very end even though Dava was too weak to respond in any way. Kay was a much-needed comfort to us that Wednesday night. She gave us hope that Dava was indeed hearing us, yet it was difficult for the girls and me to just watch her breathing and still not have her with us in the living moment. We were still praying and hoping she would open her eyes and speak. Kay did add one other note about Dava's situation that captured all of our attention when she said, "Dava is in charge now, and she might give up her spirit during the night to make it easier on us, or she might know who she wants present when she passes." Kay truly believed Dava was in control, and we were now convinced as well. As Kay left us that night, the girls and I thanked her for her gentleness and kindness with Dava and for sharing her knowledge of the situation we faced. And what Kay had conveyed to us did come to pass.

After Kay's visit, I remember having the feeling that Dava would connect with us in some manner. Even though she was unconscious, I truly did believe that she was in charge. Still, it was difficult for all of us to be lying so close and wondering if she felt our presence. That Wednesday night we all again took our turns lying on the bed next to Dava as she slept through the night. When morning arrived, Dava remained very much the same as she had been since Tuesday afternoon. Dr. Phillips came by early that morning; after greeting us and checking Dava, he shook his head from side to side and again repeated, "There is nothing wrong with her heart," only he appeared even more impressed by her strength of will. He simply added, "She's amazing!"

Andrea's short December 4th journal entry reads, *"Heart Rate – 135 / Blood Pressure – Not Readable / Breaths Per Minute – 31."* It was again the 4th of the month, and December 4th will forever remain as that immortal date imprinted on our family's hearts and souls, for Dava would not make it through to the end of the day. The room was full with the girls and me, the grandkids, brothers, sisters, sisters-in-law, and Dava's aunt and uncle. As the nurse checked Dava's vitals, all of us present heard the one reading that seemed particularly alarming, her blood pressure. It was 60 over 38. She was breathing the same steady breath of the past forty-eight hours, but the descending blood pressure was an indicator that her system was shutting down. While everyone was quietly conversing, our daughter, Sarah, spoke out in a clear and resounding tone, "I think we all need to clear out and let Dad be alone with Mom for a while." Soon the room was emptied, and again it was just "me and my honey" as Dava liked to say.

Being alone with Dava at that moment in our journey was an overwhelming experience that I will forever thank my daughters for seeing the necessity and value for our having this time together alone. I leaned very close to her, almost cheek to cheek to talk with her, to express my deep, abiding love for her, the sadness of her leaving me, and the gratefulness for her sharing her life with me these past forty-four years. I kissed her face over and over again, and my heart ached knowing she was beyond responding to my expressions of love for her. But maybe she was hearing me say, "I thank God for you and will thank Him till the day I join you in your paradise, and I thank Him for granting me the favor of having you share your life with me."

As I kissed her lips, I recalled what Dava had echoed often during her fourteen-month journey when she said, "When the time comes, where I'm in that final stage, I want you and the girls around my bed." When that thought entered my mind, I went to the door and told three of our daughters, Steph, Carrie, and Sarah that they and Andrea needed to join me in the room. I expressed to them their mother's feelings about all of us being around her bed. It was nearing two o'clock in the afternoon as the girls and I gathered around her bed. Kelsey, Carrie's daughter, was also present. We all extended our hands to touch Dava's body. I was standing on the left side of Dava at her head with Sarah across from me. Kelsey and Andrea were down from me, and Stephanie and Carrie joined Sarah on their mom's right side. Dava had the exact same breathing rate of the past two days. Suddenly to our amazement, just as we were all securely gathered around, her breath changed to a very slow pace, with a very deliberate exhale of air that appeared to curve her lips into a blowing shape. I immediately looked toward Sarah. We stared at each other for just a split second, then we all watched as Dava took five slow breaths, inhaling, then exhaling. I could hear the breath as she exhaled; and while doing so on her fifth breath, everything ceased, with her lips stopping much like a machine when the plug is pulled from its power source. It was the most graceful way one could have met death. There was no struggle, almost as if she gave out five "I love yous." I spoke first declaring, "That was the most beautiful and graceful passing anyone could have witnessed." My granddaughter, Kelsey, was crying and said, "No Grandpa, it's very sad." This moment of Dava's passing seemed so effortless, timely, and beautiful; after the fourteen months of suffering and torment, this is what she deserved and what I had hoped for her.

Andrea hurried to the nurse's station and informed the staff that her mom had stopped breathing. A doctor soon followed her back to the room. He listened for a heartbeat or pulse and then looked up, shook his head in agreement. Dava had passed. He glanced at the clock to write down the time. It was 2:10 p m on Thursday, December 4, 2008. One of the first things that came to my mind was what my cousin, Kay, had said about Dava being in charge. When Carrie and Sarah had made it known that their mom and I should have some time alone, they were not aware that

Dava had expressed her desire to have all of us around her bed. And as soon as we were all gathered, she began the process of giving up her spirit with quiet breaths, jetting upward to their heavenly journey.

Now Dava left us really wandering in the desert, for she was in her eternal sleep simply lying there. I think we were all feeling a bit lost. The nurses were very considerate and gave us time to reflect and look upon Dava before they informed us that it was time we took the next step in this journey. Then in a ragged state, we relinquished Room 7707 and said our last goodbyes, groaning and glancing back, before the door shut off the view of our beloved. In the twinkling of an eye, we were all changed. Once we had a wife, a mother, grandmother, daughter, sister, sister-in-law; now we had only the memories of each. Shakespeare's couplet to his Sonnet #50 sums up this day of remembrance:

"For that same groan doth put this in my mind
My grief lies onward and my joy behind."

I placed a call to my sister, Mary Lee, who had been through so much with us and gave her the news that Dava had passed. I then called Dava's mom and dad who were not able to be at the hospital and told them that Dava had passed peacefully just minutes before. They were deeply saddened. Some of my brothers and sisters-in-law were at the hospital and said they would inform the rest of the family. And as everyone was parting, I was wondering, so what do I do now? Half of me was staying, and I was to go home.

The ride home was almost like the mysterious one Dava and I experienced after her initial diagnosis, for I have no recollection of the afternoon or evening of Thursday, December 4th after leaving the hospital. I later sought answers from the girls, and each one remembered exactly, each one the same. We had driven two separate vehicles to my house and arrived about four o'clock. I must have been in somewhat of a trance, but the girls insist that they all wanted to read from their mother's journal and view from the picture box all of their mom's photos. Did we eat? Did we have an appetite to eat? I doubt we had anything but a longing to somehow come to grips with our loss. The one word that best describes our grief that evening we spent together would be heartbroken, yet as the evening progressed, we adopted more comforting and loving expressions as our loved one, Dava, would have wanted. No one mentioned sleep. How one sleeps after a day we had all lived through can only be explained by the fact that we were overcome with exhaustion.

We watched our loved one's every breath, especially those final five; and part of this day vanished with those breaths to where we had nothing left, no fresh air to breathe. The day was done; all we could do now was exist. It's hard, very hard, to lose someone so close. We will remember Dava every day of our lives. Spouses and their children have this incredible bond. Once it is shattered, the heart will never completely heal.

My daughter Carrie spent the night at my place because she did not think I should have to spend this first night all alone. She said that she awoke two or three times during the night thinking this day was all a dreadful dream. Maybe I fell asleep just because I was exhausted with nothing else to do; and maybe I could visit Dava in a dream which has been my desire to this day. So this ended the final day of Dava's life on this earth, but our hearts carry her with us each and every day forever.

chapter nineteen

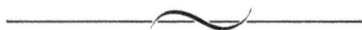

Dava's Memorial and Funeral

If I had been able to totally view Dava's passing in objective reality, maybe I could have more easily accepted it and had a sense of relief; after all, Dava was no longer having to suffer. But now that she was gone, I realized how really difficult it was to have lost the love of my life. I had never actually contemplated losing her at all; until the hour of her passing, she was my strength throughout her long and arduous journey of fighting the cancer.

All along there was the knowledge that this type of cancer was so deadly that more than ninety-five percent perish in the first two years, and the biggest percentage die within a few months of diagnosis. I can still feel the shock to my system when Dr. Van Amburg told me that he didn't think Dava would make it through the day on that Tuesday. However, there were reasons for that news to be shocking when I think back three and a half weeks earlier before the throwing up of blood when Dava had some decent, good days where she smiled and laughed, when we were trying to make this life somewhat normal. But the loss of blood was too much; her life's blood was literally draining daily the little energy she had left to fight on. This was all happening right in front of me, but I still thought this wasn't going to end here, that she would get better and carry on the fight until the day came where the cancer conquered her. Nevertheless, I think I will always live the rest of my days shocked that she is no longer with me. I guess I didn't realize that the shock would never ever leave, and yet I cherish it as a reminder of our love for one another.

On Friday morning December 5th, I awoke still in somewhat of a trance, not sure of my next step. There was to be a meeting this day at the funeral home which was scheduled at eleven o'clock for the girls and me to attend. Before that meeting, I called my nephew, Father Mitch Doyen, about presiding at Dava's funeral service at St. Rose of Lima Church in De Soto. He was most gracious in his accepting as he had been many times in the past for family. I also contacted two singers, Aaron Hardin and Janet Vilmer, to do the singing. We planned some of the customary funeral hymns, but I also requested they sing the song Dava had brought to my attention months earlier, "Your Long Journey," that last number on the album, *Raising Sand*. One last thing I did that morning was to contact my sister

Judy and my brother Rob to ask them to speak of Dava toward the end of the service. They both agreed. With these important functions taken care of, I just waited to head to the funeral home with Carrie to join her sisters and the funeral director.

The five of us sat around a table with Jake, the owner of Dietrich–Mothershead Funeral Home in De Soto. Jake was very professional and made it easy for us in all our decisions and planning. One question Jake asked was concerning the type vault, the basic one for $600.00 or the Titan vault for $1295.00; before I could think or answer, Sarah said, "Dad, you are getting Mom the better vault," to which I answered, "Yes, we are." The remainder of our meeting consisted of setting the date and time for funeral home visitation on Sunday December 7th, 3 p.m. to 8 p.m. and the funeral at St. Rose of Lima on Monday morning December 8th. After the meeting, I returned home to just sit and meditate. One of the girls, still thinking I shouldn't be alone, came out later that evening to spend the night.

Of all the days immediately following Dava's passing that I coveted the most was Saturday, for there was nothing on the agenda. My total thoughts that day were on Dava and dealing with my grief. Late that morning my sister Judy called and asked if maybe I needed to get anything, like a suit or shoes, etc. I emphasized that most of all I needed time alone, but after some thought, I decided that a new suit would be nice if I could go and not spend time shopping, just pick one out and return home. Judy assured me that she and Mark would take me to pick out a suit and be back in the shortest amount of time. I recall going to Macy's, standing in the dressing room after giving Mark my sizes. He would hand me three or four without a word until one fit to perfection, a black suit. Judy meanwhile gathered up a white shirt and tie, and we were heading back to my house, or is it still our house? I began to see there was a lot to learn and get used to, and I wasn't sure how to say everything yet. It was a little over two hours, mostly on the road, and we were done, just like Mark and Judy said.

So Saturday afternoon I returned to my living room and sat wanting to think only of Dava, but I needed to contact Dava's parents to let them know all the details about upcoming events. Her dad thought a Sunday night visitation was a bad idea because he said it was a church night for Baptists. I informed David that the funeral director suggested that date which is the third day after the death when visitations are normally held. He graciously said it was my wish and thought everything was fine. I again mentioned that there would be many visitors who knew Dava and her family. The rest of Saturday I spent in mourning. My heart was broken, and my thoughts were of Dava; I wept. Later that evening, one of the girls came to spend the night.

During the first hour of the visitation, our immediate family assembled in front of Dava's coffin. In our eyes, she was a Sleeping Beauty though the essence of her being was not there. It was Dava and yet it was not, but that's what death is all about, removing the essence of being from that beautiful person lying there before us. Dava often chided me that my funeral visitation would garner nearly everyone in town whereas she would more than likely have only a handful for herself. But she misjudged this night, for the visitors kept coming for the full four hours to pay their respects. Over six hundred people passed through to view her for the last time. It was not the number that mattered; it was the love expressed for her among the many family and friends. As sad as the evening was, the fact that those in line waited thirty to forty minutes to offer their condolences and to let us know they shared in our sorrow was a testament to Dava and all her family and friends. The experience was humbling and at the same time enlightening. I was the last to leave the room that night. I kissed my beloved on her lips and said goodbye again. Since the girls thought I needed company, one of them spent the night at the house.

The funeral Mass the next morning was both heartwarming and heartbreaking at the same time. Fr. Mitch's talk was filled with fond memories of his Aunt Dava and inspiring and compassionate words to help us deal with our loss. Rob quoted Shakespeare's Sonnet 116 and related it to Dava's love for us and our love for her. Then Judy spoke of her closeness to Dava, especially during her teen years, and the love that Dava engendered in abundance. My brother Charlie played guitar for the final song, "Your Long Journey," as Aaron and Janet sang. The song struck me and the girls like an arrow to the heart. It was so meaningful and such a beautiful way to end the funeral service that left us in tears and total tranquility.

The graveside ceremony almost escaped one's thinking because it appeared so unseemly to even think of leaving a loved one alone to await the darkness of night. But we did what had to be done and departed for a gathering at the Knights of Columbus Hall to nourish our bodies, but more importantly, to share with those who were there to comfort us. After the food and socializing, it was time to go home alone, realizing I would never be able to see Dava's face again; such thoughts of living without her began to haunt my spirit again.

chapter twenty

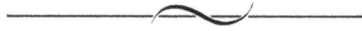

Learning to Live Life
With Dava's Spirit at My Side

From this point to the end of the narrative, I will dwell more on my feelings and experiences and the girls' future endeavors that Dava influenced to a great degree. Though she is gone in body, her spirit remains among us. It may appear to some an insignificant matter, but the girls within days of losing their mother began noticing "smiley faces" appearing here and there. After a time, they started to wonder: is this some sign that their mom was near? Truly amazing images of "smiley faces" showed up in all sorts of places, maybe in a footprint in the snow, or a lot of times in foods or liquids, or the face in a pizza with perfect eyes, nose, and a smile. Every time one appeared, one of the girls would text what she saw to the rest of us. I soon became a believer myself.

The girls did inform me that this phenomenon was not general knowledge, that it was known only among the family. Others would not understand without a full explanation. It is quite amazing how many hundreds of "smiley faces" have shown up over the past ten years. Dava has not gone too far from us.

One of the first things I did personally was to attend St. Xavier College Church at St. Louis University for Sunday Mass. It's about an hour's drive from De Soto, but it was well worth the trip to hear their very talented choir. After experiencing the magnificence of the choir during their Christmas celebrations, I was fortunate enough to join this choir for six months, and it proved to be something I needed in that period of my life. I felt grateful to the music director and choir members for allowing me the honor of singing with them. They ended up helping me much more than I helped them, and I will never forget the many benefits this experience provided as an outlet during a difficult time.

My daughters had worked out a rotation schedule of staying with me night after night for about eight or nine days after Dava passed. On the following Friday, Carrie called me to say that she didn't think anyone could make it that night, and she was worried about me. I let her know that I always enjoyed having any or all of my girls around, but I was fine being alone. I assured her that there was no need to keep up the nightly stayovers; I had no problem being here alone, and they all had tough enough schedules in their lives these days to manage. I added that it was nice having someone around who was hurting as much as I was hurting but being alone was something I would get used to, and eventually everything would be fine. It was so very kind of them to be so concerned with my well-being, and I will always be grateful for their thoughtfulness.

On the 20th of December, I received a Christmas card to both Dava and me from Bonnie and Mike. Bonnie was the kind and generous lady who allowed Dava to take her turn in receiving her radiation treatment. My heart saddened immediately on receiving their card; for a few seconds, I caught myself desiring their state of not knowing. In their minds Dava still lived. After a few minutes of letting myself imagine that we were both here to read the card, I called their number and Bonnie answered. After I mentioned receiving the Christmas card, I realized that they were not aware that Dava had passed away in early December. Bonnie was so kind and generous with her words that it was indeed a blessing and a comfort to speak with her. She spoke about how beautiful Dava was and that she would be thinking of me and the girls. I thanked her for entering our lives and especially in the way she did by giving up her place in line to help Dava.

We agreed to meet sometime in the future. Later in February, my sister Mary Lee and I met Bonnie and Mike for lunch. I will always remember these very special people.

One kind act turned into a beautiful friendship and a great memory of ten years for me.

As everyone knows, the holiday season can bring on additional feelings of melancholy after the loss of a loved one. The first Christmas brought forth a torrent of tears with thoughts of our previous times together. It had been only three weeks between Dava's passing and Christmas, but that may have helped us heal. This time of year is such a close time for family gatherings and sharing memories, and Dava gave us countless numbers of them to recall. We made Christmas the best that we could with the girls and grandkids gathering on Christmas Eve as we had been doing every year. I could almost picture Dava looking in our living room window that night with the angels as her escort saying, "Thank You Lord, they are together, one and all, and there is so much love gathered among them, and I do so love them, each and every one." We were all hurting deeply but managed to have our Christmas as Dava would have wished.

Andrea was so saddened with this being the first Christmas without her Mom, she waited till December 28th to make this entry in her journal:

"Mom died that day, Dec. 4th, 2008 at 2:10 p m. I haven't written since that day, which was about thirty minutes before she passed. What a sad day, what a sad week, now nearing a

sad month. We all had slept and sat around Mom Sunday through Thursday, she somewhat realized we were there that Tuesday, but couldn't show it after that, in and out of her dazes, in and out with the morphine. Tuesday her room was surrounded with people, packed, we all thought she wouldn't make it through the day. Wednesday her breathing was about the same (12 to 15 breaths a minute). She was too high on the morphine to move by then.

"Kelsey and I decided to bathe her. I washed her hair, Kelsey filed her nails, I flossed her teeth. We had the nurses move her around, reposition her – She was much better and more comfortable. I hope she knew we were doing it. I knew Mom didn't want to "smell like a donkey" as she would always say.

"Thursday we were all awake and semi ready for another day in the hospital. I even asked Kelsey if she wanted to go to the nearby mall – thank goodness we didn't. Mom's breathing was getting faster – (30 to 38) times a minute, like she was running a race (a race with death). Sarah had the nurse come in around 1:30 p m to check her vitals – they couldn't even get her blood pressure reading. Sarah thought Dad needed some time alone w/ Mom. About 2: 05 Dad called us back in. Steph, Carrie, Sarah, and Kelsey went in w/ him – he sent for me. I was in the waiting room, and John and Onie asked if I wanted to go to the Bistro Cafe in the hospital. I told them I'd meet them a little later down there, that I was going back to Mom's room. Everyone in our little family was gathering around her bed – I was at her left side by her feet. She began breathing slowly again, very slow. I mentioned her face and lips were very white. She took 5 slow last breaths and she was gone. Her mouth open – I remember Dad just saying, " Oh," so sadly and we all cried. We said the "Our Father" around her. I went out and told the nurses, they all began to cry – I really think they felt something for Mom and our family.

"We packed up and went to Dad's that night – looking through the pictures. The visitation was Sunday, it was amazing – non stop, until 8 PM – you feel the love in the room. And the funeral on Monday morning was beautiful. Just as Mom would have wanted. I miss her bad – I think of her daily, hourly in fact. I wonder about her thoughts those last couple of days that she wasn't able to talk – did she hear all the times I whispered "I love you" in her ear – does she realize the love we all have for her and what she did and meant to us?

"That Monday before she died, she called us all around her bed side – she even sat up, she told us all how much she loved us all, and that she couldn't take it anymore, and she did not want to go home to hospice. It was a good night, I only wish I had known it was our last night that she could talk to us. I would have said so much more. The kids have taken it hard. Ethan doesn't fully understand being only 3 and 1/2, Emily does. She shed a lot of tears, and does miss her Granny.

She sleeps in Granny's robe every night, and looks for the brightest star at night looking for Granny. They visit the cemetery and Ethan talks and prays to Granny. It will be rough for all of us – but Mom isn't suffering – although I know she's in a better place. I didn't say much – I remember Mom saying she didn't want people looking at her and saying, "Oh, she's in a better place." Though we know she's with God, she would love to still be at home and I wish she was, I miss & love you Mom. Good night."

I have tried to cover all the aspects of this journey, but I have avoided for the most part its lasting effects on me. I was lost, and I had many others looking out for me. The girls checked on me several times each day at the beginning, especially if they had not heard from me or for some reason couldn't reach me. The hurt at times was so severe, it seemed that every thought of Dava made me ten times sadder than I already was, and yet, for some inexplicable reason, I wanted to be taken down to the very depths where the grief gave way to crying to relieve some of the hurt. At times I could almost hear her speak to me. It was forty-four years of togetherness, and now the covenant had been breached, broken, and smashed; nevertheless, my love for Dava grew to new heights. It now seemed to me she was on a higher plain which I couldn't reach or comprehend. While she was still with me, we shared nearly everything whereas now she knows so much more about the secrets of the world that are still unknown to me. No one knows with absolute certainty what lies ahead of us after death, but I do know my intense desire to touch, to talk. and tell Dava how much I love her and that she has increased my yearning for everlasting life and made it my everlasting plea. One moment with her now would exceed any other desire I have on this earth. If that sounds extreme, and it might for those who have not experienced such a personal loss as this, it isn't when one considers that I have had ten years to prepare for such a short encounter; and the love I would show her and receive back tenfold would hold for all eternity.

It was the month of January with the holiday festivities behind me when the darkest hours approached. The barren blast of winter was with us, not just in body, but also in our souls. It was a day this month that Patrick Swayze was featured on the *Barbara Walters Special*, and I so wished that Dava had had the opportunity to see him. He had been diagnosed with pancreatic cancer just a few months after Dava's. I knew that he knew he wasn't going to survive the cancer. He was amazing in his explanation of this terrifying disease, saying everything Dava and I felt in holding up the helpless hope that we also hung on to so tenaciously. He had been fighting the cancer for eleven months, and he was prepared for the worst which would come nine months later. I just wish we would have connected with him back in

February of 2008. Dava and I felt the connection the minute we heard he had the disease, and I think we could have possibly helped each other. I could have empathized with his wife, Lisa, and the feelings that were consuming her; Dava would have connected with Patrick in sharing their common bond in fighting such a deadly cancer. It may seem like a stretch to imagine such exchanges, but in the end, we are all just human beings needing each other in our times of need. I'm sure that our meeting and communicating would have helped us.

In February 2009 I had seen a notice for singers for the Jefferson College Adult Choir. The following Tuesday I went to the college only to find out the choir had already begun rehearsals the week before, but after explaining my recent loss and circumstances, the music director was very accommodating and agreed to let me participate. That evening he gave me a disc of the music being rehearsed which was John Rutter's *Requiem*, plus *The Lord Is My Shepherd* selections. As I sat in my darkened living room listening to this glorious music, my heart began to speed up with all the emotions swelling up inside of me. I had written in my journal later in the week about this very spiritual experience. My journal entry from February 2009:

"Since Tuesday, Dava has been on my mind non-stop, mainly due to my listening to Rutter's Requiem and The Lord is my Shepherd recordings. I rehearsed with the college chorus, but

the disc that was given to me has been such a blessing to where I feel I was somehow guided to what I did. It revealed to me what I thought Dava was going through those last two days when she was unable to communicate with us. I know the girls wondered what their Mom was thinking as she lay there, just breathing, no, not just breathing, more than likely she knew everything that was going on, but didn't have the physical strength to share her thoughts with us. I believe Dava realized she was leaving us and she was aware that there were no words in our vocabulary that could express her love for us more deeply than she had shown us in her life. And her deep sadness at leaving us behind is beyond words also; Dava had given us all she had to give and there simply was no more for her to do or say. What a blessing to have had her in our lives for as long as we did, and the girls and grandkids have her bloodline which is even a greater gift. She is so loved by everyone and I am so sad to be alone, although that's a selfish thing to note, but my heart is nearly breaking and I don't want it to break, so I'll have to live with the extreme loneliness that comes at times and this I can't fully explain. I love you."

Andrea's journal entry of January 4th, 2009, exactly one month since her mother's passing:

"One month since Mom passed away. I think of her often, I miss her so. Is it selfish of me to want her back, even in the

shape she was in just for that Monday before she died, to talk more with her, to lay with her longer, to let her know the love we all have for her? I still watch the video made for the funeral visitations made for her, over and over – I just watched it last night alone, cried the whole way through and watched it twice with Dad and with Emily tonight. Goodnight Mom. p.s. Em showed me the brightest star tonight, she looks for you every night in the brightest star. She talks about you every day – but you know that. Ethan asked Dad tonight when you're coming home – I know God took you for a reason, but I want you back here so bad. I love you Mom.

Andrea wrote another journal entry on January 26th, 2009:

"At my adoration hour, Sarah came with me tonight. We joined Weight Watchers and Snap Fitness together. Stayed at Dad's with the kids last night --- Mick and Dad came to get us, I had sold my van yesterday. I am now driving Mom's Jeep – I know she didn't get to drive it much, but it was part of her and I wanted it, I do love it. Tonight I made hamburgers, pretty good I might add, and we all watched Patrick Swayze and Barbara Walters interview again – I think I've seen it about six times now. I don't mind, it's kinda like watching Mom's video, you never get tired of watching it. I do miss her awfully bad and think of her a dozen times a day. I usually hide my tears, I break down on my Chapel hour, sometimes while lying in the tanning bed, or like at night while sleeping with Ethan at 2:30 am it hits me. Some days I can't believe she's gone, some days I really need her. I do find comfort going to their house, and spending time with Dad, going through Mom's things, reading her journals.

"I even went looking through her bathroom cabinets and drawers just to have memories of her smell or to just remember when we hung out in there while the kids were in the tub. I remember one day I went out, she was so frail, washing herself in the bathroom sink – she asked me to come in, she looked so pitiful, so skinny. It was so sad. I remember in those couple of months, all of us girls laying around her, watching the "Little House on the Prairie" movies with her. I think we are all ok – and we have our "moments" – and of course we all would rather have her here – it just hasn't quite sunk in w/ me that she's gone. It feels more like she left for a trip to Wal Mart, that's why she's not here – not like she's gone forever. We do look for the brightest star each night – Emily swears that's her Granny.

"Reading her journals are special, not that I ever doubted her love for us – but she spoke of her love so often. She often told me in person and in her journals that she thought I opened up more to Dad. I guess maybe I always have, but when she was sick, I didn't want her to have more to worry about. I do love my Dad, and feel very close to him and think my life would be over if I lost him too."

Andrea's journal entry on February 8, 2009:

"Went out w/the crew of friends last night – it's been 10 years since our dear friend Speedy died – I can't believe it. I hope it doesn't go that fast since Mom died. I try to talk of her often and I think of her nearly nonstop. It's Abby's birthday – Mom was always at our kids birthdays. Looking at pictures of her. I keep the ones from the hospital in my purse and glance at them a lot. The kids ask about her everyday. Emily must write "Granny" on something at least once a day. Em just ask me tonight before bed if Granny knew what she was thinking in her mind – I told her I talk to her all the time in my head – she just smiled. Ethan just wants to know when Granny's coming home! Dad seems like he's doing ok – everyone asks me everyday, how he's doing or how I'm doing. I have my kids, my work – but Dad's by himself and I hate that, Maybe he likes it that way, but I feel bad for him. Watch over him Mom, and us too."

It was sometime in early March that I began looking for our gravestone. I knew I wanted to go with a red granite to match my mom's and dad's stone. But I also wanted some saying or quotation on Dava's portion of the stone, something from a piece of literature, whether it be sacred or secular. I called two of my brothers, Rob and Mick, and asked them to give some thought as to what might be appropriate for Dava's stone. Rob returned my call with an excellent suggestion of using a Shakespeare quote from the last scene of *Hamlet*; but at the same time, I remembered the quote from Shakespeare's *Romeo and Juliet* that I settled on to adorn Dava's stone. It reads: "Her beauty makes this vault a feasting presence, full of light."

Andrea's journal entry on March 29, 2009:

"At chapel hour again – Mom is still on my mind – I was looking at pictures and all her decorating she did to her house – it's all Mom. I miss her a lot, it still feels like some days she's going to come home. Dad's been great, keeping busy singing at the college, and at St. Xavier's in St. Louis. He ordered Mom's gravestone – the kids' birthdays are in this month – Emily's a big 7, Ethan turns 4."

Andrea's journal entry on April 12, 2009, Easter Sunday:

"At my chapel hour once again – it's Easter, a very sad day w/o Mom – God, I miss her so much. Dad summed it up the other day while talking to a customer. 'Some days I think of Dava non-stop, and the others I get mad at myself because I didn't pause enough to think of her as I should.'

"The kids ask about her a lot -- Emily put on a t-shirt and commented that "Granny" ironed the "iron on" on her shirt – she said it itched but she kept it on because Granny made it. Ethan asked me tonight when Granny will come back from heaven – I told him that she's always with us here.

As the Christmas of 2009 was approaching, the girls and I knew we needed to make December 4th a very memorable date to honor the memory of Dava, my beloved wife and their mother. We decided that everything else could be set aside for us to spend this day together in joy, fun, happiness, and reflection. We met that first anniversary at Dava's grave site to announce that this was the day of remembrance of her; and after a few words and prayers, we climbed into one vehicle and headed to West County Shopping Mall in St. Louis County. The conversations during the ride there were mostly reflections on how their mom and the girls spent hours shopping before Christmas.

We first stopped at Macy's where I told the girls to pick out the perfume of their choice. It was fun for me to watch as each one searched and tested to find her favorite fragrance. The shopping at Macy's was followed by a late afternoon dinner at the California Pizza Kitchen where again we shared more Mom stories. Then they left in pairs for more shopping, and I alone went to the men's area to look around a bit myself. By the time we finally gathered near 8 PM for some dessert, I was ready to call it a wonderful day, and the girls graciously gave up their shopping. On the way home, we were all in a happy mood; and I even suggested singing a song or two. All in all, it was a perfect way to remember Dava's Anniversary.

So now it is ten years hence, and just yesterday evening,

December 1, 2018, we did very much the exact same thing for the tenth time. The ladies at the perfume counter at Macy's even recognized us, and several knew the story of why we are there every year on the Saturday just before December 4th. What is so special about this day for me is the fact that this would have been a day Dava would have loved being with us. Such a time would compare to those long shopping days during the holidays. I look forward to this event more than any throughout the year, but it wouldn't mean anything to any of us if Dava wasn't at the center of the day.

chapter twenty-one

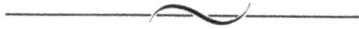

Reunion of Remembrances

It was the following year of 2010 that there was a family reunion planned over the 4th of July weekend. It was to be held in St. Louis, and I knew I wanted to honor Dava's absence in some way. It wasn't till I began reading Whitman's Leaves of Grass that the perfect, literary work presented itself to me. It was Whitman's farewell address to his lover as he prepared for his own death. The poem appealed to me after the first reading; and I wanted to read it at the reunion; but after several readings, I realized I needed to reply to what I considered my Fancy speaking to me. So I finally decided I not only would read Whitman's "Goodbye My Fancy" but also read my reply to it. After reading the poem over and over, it began speaking to me of the feelings of one departing this life, and I couldn't leave its impact dangling without answering a lover's departing goodbye. Whitman's poem reads as follows:

Reunion of Remembrances

"Good-Bye My Fancy!"

Good-bye my Fancy!

Farewell dear mate, dear love!

I'm going away, I know not where,

Or to what fortune, or whether I may ever see you again,

So Good-bye my Fancy.

Now for my last – let me look back a moment;

The slower fainter ticking of the clock is in me,

Exit, nightfall, and soon the heart-thud stopping.

Long have we lived, joy'd, caress'd together;

Delightful! – now separation – Good-bye my Fancy.

Yet let me not be too hasty,

Long indeed have we lived, slept, filter'd, become really blended into one;

Then if we die we die together, (yes, we'll remain one,)

If we go anywhere we'll go together to meet what happens,

May-be we'll be better off and blither, and learn something,

May-be it is yourself now really ushering me to the true songs, (who knows?)

May-be it is you the mortal knob really undoing, turning – so now finally,

Good-bye – and hail! my Fancy.

I wrote my reply to this thought-provoking poem in prose, and my brother, Mick, took my words and arranged them in poetic free verse:

In Reply to Whitman's

"Good-Bye My Fancy!"

Two years ago, this very day

We huddled together, you and I,

As you suffered so courageously

With the pains of the cancer.

Our thoughts were with the family

Reunion of Remembrances

Celebrating a reunion miles away

And you kept insisting I take part;

And you in your selfless nature

Knew so much better than I that

This was where I needed to be and

Wanted to be, with you, my Fancy.

Now I realize in retrospect

Just how much I needed you;

How I could never get enough of you,

Why I should have kissed you

A few more times those final days

And never let go of you, my Fancy.

Your beautiful eyes, your enduring smile

That these plain eyes ever eyed.

Oh what beauty God gave me in you!

In my seeking, somehow I found you,

My sweet, my darling, my Dava,

My Fancy then, and now, and forever.

In this your birthday month, my love,

I can not help but feel

That you left us much too soon.

But for some reason unknown to us

God decided that your beauty,

Sweet Fancy, should be with Him.

So goodbye, my Fancy,

Know that my longings are for you

And your eternal happiness,

And my desire to one day be with you.

My heart fills with love

At the very thought of you.

Everything I wanted to say to Dava on that final day I wanted to express in my reply. Whitman's poem provided a world of emotions for me with words like, "I'm going away, I know not where, or to what fortune, or whether I may ever see you again." How profound and succinct is the sublime surrender that seems to sever the oneness of our souls. And then comes the beautiful line expressing oneness: "Then if we die we die together, (yes, we'll remain one)." The first half of this line reminds me of Romeo's and Juliet's desire fulfilled, and yet if one lives, we will still remain as one. There is so much meaning for me throughout this generous, gentle, and emotionally charged poem, and I felt compelled to reply with words that expressed my deepest feelings within my being to make the goodbye bearable.

chapter twenty-two

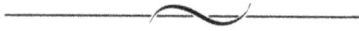

Touched by a Hand

When people reflect on particular instances in their lives, maybe it would be safe to say that there might very well be an incident of such significance that a person could imagine or think there was some miraculous intervention involved. One such incident occurred in my life on an evening in the month of May 2014 after sharing a meal with family at my sister Mary Lee's place. I left the house about 6:30 to attend choir practice at Our Lady's Parish in Festus which is about fourteen miles from De Soto.

It was raining as it had been doing most of the day. I was cruising Highway 67 doing sixty miles an hour in the right lane of a four-lane highway. U S Highway 67 with two lanes in both directions is definitely one of the older roads dating back to the forties when it was the main expressway to St. Louis. With no concerns and singing along with music on the radio, I was suddenly shocked to attention when my car suddenly began hydroplaning. At first for just seconds, it seemed as though the car was floating before I found my-self going sideways down the highway. There was no time for prayers or planning. All that was running through my mind was that this was going to be bad.

After sliding maybe a hundred yards sideways, the ve-hicle went forcefully into the grassy median where it was spinning in circles with grass and mud splashing against the windshield. Then it traveled another seventy yards backwards and came to a stop after completing 180 degrees near the oncoming traffic on the other side of the median. It all happened so quickly, as accidents usually do, I just sat in the car trying to collect myself and noticing I was on the shoulder facing traffic on the other side. After pulling the car a little farther away from the oncoming traffic, I began thinking how and why I made it through this harrowing experience in one piece.

Just by coincidence, my daughter Carrie and her hus-band Mike were on the same highway about five miles ahead of where I was at the time. After I placed the call to them, I stayed in the car looking over at the three-layered cable fencing connected at intervals by concrete posts in the median. After about fifteen minutes or so, Carrie and Mike arrived on the scene where they could see my car on the opposite shoulder heading the wrong way on the south-bound lanes. After surveying the scene for a few minutes, Mike informed me that my vehicle had just missed two of the concrete posts where there was a space in the cabled fencing. I surveyed the area myself and noticed the concrete posts and some large boulders covering much of the median except the small grassy area where my car had descended and traveled through to the other side. Although I was considerably shaken, I suffered no injuries. I was still quite stunned and thinking: how could one be so fortunate after spinning out of control at sixty miles per hour, facing concrete posts, some huge boulders, and cable fencing and still come out unscathed?

A young police officer arrived shortly after the incident happened and just listened to my rambling on about how I just missed the protective fencing. He informed me that the fencing was there for the protection of drivers on this side of the highway, and if I had hit the cabled fencing, he would have been calling an ambulance. After surveying the site and looking over the car, he looked at me and said, "Someone was looking out for you." He even offered to take me to choir practice since my car was stuck in the mud. I graciously thanked him for coming by and said I was heading home after I called a wrecker to retrieve my car from the mud.

Why speak of this incident in my story? Well, just maybe someone *was looking* out for me. I still shiver at times when I think back on those precarious few seconds of that episode in my life. Carrie once suggested that Mom didn't want us kids to be orphans. Whatever the case, twelve days later sitting alone at home reflecting on this experience, the thought that Dava may have had a hand in the outcome prompted me to write on 5-26-14 this testimony which I refer to as "Touched by a Hand:"

"Who would have thought after a meal with my sister and brothers what fate lay in store for me? But an event occurred that may well have taken me out of existence or left me in dire circumstances, for the water was in control, and I wasn't, no matter my diligence at the time. In not minutes but seconds, and very few of them, I was led to a place of peril. Suddenly in the twinkling of an eye, I was tossed in every direction, sideways, backwards, and twisting with my only concern to prepare for the worse and brace myself. Eight seconds is what a bull rider rides to glory; and in that mode, I'm hanging on for life, and finally it comes to an end. I rest, realizing the eight seconds are over, and I am unhurt and not even much damage I can see. But how and why am I still intact? I was traveling at 60 mph and shooting out of the hydroplaning at 70 mph, not in control and preparing for the worst. I am whole. Then I imagine myself emerging from the median into the path of oncoming traffic or hitting the cabled fencing or one of the concrete poles. No, I missed all obstacles, but only by inches. I truly believe Dava's hands were not only on me, but her arms were around me. Why? I do not know. The future may reveal it to me. I was too shocked and frightened

to think of why then but not now. I can picture Dava pleading my case; the only reason I can offer is her love for me, and I will never take it for granted! Love from the one who felt the touch of your hand, G D."

chapter twenty-three

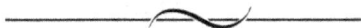

The Moon Beams a Solemn Night

It was a cold wintry night in late January as I sat reading and listening to some beautiful music. With a bourbon drink in hand, I grabbed my coat and went outside on my upper deck to breathe in the brisk winter wind.

I searched the skies, but the grayish clouds, brightened by the hidden moon, were rolling by when in an instant the glorious, bright, full moon appeared dead center in the southern sky. It was so crisp and bright I couldn't take my eyes off its glow, and soon thoughts of Dava speaking to me took control. And for some moments, we were communicating back and forth; and just as suddenly as that full moon appeared, it disappeared just as quickly with the graying clouds swarming over it. I was drained of an energy I had just had, and I felt a cold chill set in and reentered the house. I went to bed thinking about that visitation and awoke the next morning with the exact same, intense feeling. I wrote this poem because the vision of that night was still there.

"Solemn Night"

One night gazing upward the full moon
Masked by the graying clouds became bright.
Awakened memories vanquished soon
Ev'ry thought 'cept her this wintry night.

Though bitter cold while seeming so warm
Looking deeper into the orb's glow,
Visions came of her clothed in my arms
Her beauty beckoning this should be so.

In the midst of joyous tranquility
Mournful clouds in all directions formed
The loss of all sensibility
As though my mind and heart were disjoined.

Moments passed, the orb's light disappeared
Eyes affixed on the darkness beyond.
My fancy's fate realized, I feared,
Allowed one last gasp, my God, she's gone.

G D. 1-30-15

Remembrances and memories are what we have left of our lives with Dava, and I feel I have a responsibility to keep her alive in our minds and hearts. This I try to do with anyone I come into contact with when discussing all that really matters to me. She is on my mind daily, not to the point of distraction from other endeavors, but I feel her spirit is but a breath away. Asking her for help and guidance seems so natural for me that it is done without deliberate forethought, for it's easier to simply say, "Dava, show me the way." Sometimes I want to say , "I'm sorry" that life put her through those painful and trying times, but again, it's much easier to say, "I love you."

chapter twenty-four

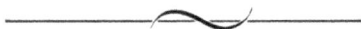

Close

If I were to have to eliminate from memory any ten-year period of Dava and my life together, it would be impossible for me to do. That would create a vast vacuum in our journey toward our togetherness, and it would be simply too painful to consider. To erase from my mind any ten-year period without Dava is too difficult, yet I have lived through ten years since her death without her.

To begin those first ten years of marriage from 1968 to 1978 were more than enchanting. Even going back to 1964 when we first met and started dating, I can recall nearly every moment of these first times together. Through our dating years when just having her near me was heavenly, those early steps that we took together kept us growing closer and closer as we fell in love with one another. We married in 1968 and had all four of our daughters within these ten years. We were a budding family and already a close-knit family. There is no way I would give these ten years back.

The next set of ten years from 1978 to 1988 were the years where we found that true love was picking one another up on those rough days and making the most of our special times together to where it would really mean something to both of us. I recall our girls making friends, and their friends loved coming to our home. It was not just another house to visit but a home where they found love existing there; and I recall years later some expressed their feelings of the love and family togetherness they found there in letters and cards to Dava, the girls, and me. No way I'd trade these ten years for anything.

During the following ten years from 1988 to 1998, two of our daughters were married, and we discovered the joys of having grandchildren. Our family remained close, not only in distance but in keeping in contact with one another almost on a daily basis. Traditions that were formed from earlier times were solidified, and the continuance of those traditions like our Christmas Eve get-togethers made the memories even more memorable. No way I would let these ten years slip away.

Then comes our last ten years together from 1998 to 2008 when the younger two girls were married, and more grandchildren followed. These were the years when Dava and I for the most part lived alone in our home, but it sure didn't seem like we were missing out on anything. We were on a new adventure, the two of us, and just enjoying each other to the fullest; we cherished our evenings alone together. Then came the cancer diagnosis that attempted to turn our lives upside down, and at times one could say it succeeded. The fourteen months of dealing with pancreatic cancer, when faced with one tragic event after another, our love for each other developed into the deepest love that ever existed in our lives. Throughout our never-ending struggles, we were wanting so much to hang on to each other every moment for as long as we could. No way I would ever consider giving up these ten years either.

Many of these last ten years from 2008 to 2018 for me were spent reflecting on the previous sets of ten, often I might add. I have had plenty of time to think of all the ways having Dava in my life made me a better person, and I think she would agree that I helped her be a better person too. It's possible that I may have been able to have had a love relationship without Dava that endured for forty years, but I wouldn't have wanted to gamble on it. You see, I sort of felt like I hit the jackpot and was the more fortunate one to have had Dava as my mate.

So I can't have it both ways, to be satisfied with my good fortune in having my darling Dava through forty, precious years of life with me, and then wonder why fortune failed me, leaving me alone without her. As I once again recall Keats' poem, "Welcome Joy, Welcome Sorrow," where he considered both joy and sorrow as existing together as one. I have joyfully accepted the joy, so the same must be with sorrow. I would never give up the sorrow to not have experienced such joy, no way.

Appendix

Quotations related to pancreatic cancer and death.

Excerpts from *The Emperor of All Maladies*
by Siddhartha Mukherjee:

"Recall Atossa, the Persian queen who likely had breast cancer in 500 B C . . . She will likely take some form of medicine, whether to prevent, cure, or palliate her illness for the rest of her life.

"This indubitably is progress. But before we become too dazzled by Atossa's survival, it is worthwhile putting it into perspective. Give Atossa metastatic pancreatic cancer in 500 B C and her prognosis is unlikely to change by more than a few months over twenty-five hundred years." (pages 463 and 465)

"Cancer therapy is like beating the dog with a stick to get rid of the fleas," by Anna Deavere Smith, from "Let Me Down Easy," as quoted in Mukherjee's *The Emperor of All Maladies*. (page 305)

"Even in oncology, a dismal discipline to begin with, this—unresected pancreatic cancer—was considered the epitome of the dismal.

"Sorensen's life had turned upside down. 'I want to beat it to the end.' She told me at first . . . We blasted her pancreas with radiation, followed with chemotherapy. The tumor had grown right through all the treatments. We switched to a new drug, Gemzar . . . 'She will try anything, anything,' her husband pleaded. 'She is stronger than she looks.'

"Beatrice finally broke the awkward silence. 'I'm sorry.' She shrugged her shoulders and looked vacantly past us, 'I know we have reached an end.'

"We hung our heads, ashamed. It was, I suspected, not the first time that a patient had consoled a doctor about the ineffectuality of his discipline." (page 154)

From the Last Scene of *Death of a Salesman*
by Arthur Miller:

"I search and search and I search, and I can't understand it, Willy. I made the last payment on the house today. Today, dear. And there'll be nobody home. We're free and clear. We're free . . . We're free . . ."

From the book, *The Art of Death*,
by Elwidge Danticat:

Appendix

"As the father of the essay, Michel de Montaigne, writes, 'Dying . . . is the greatest work we have to do,' "yet we can't get good at it by practicing, since we experience it only once."

And from this same source, Simone de Beauvoir is quoted as saying from her book, *A Very Easy Death:* "You do not die from being born, nor from having lived, nor from old age. You die from something . . . cancer, thrombosis, pneumonia: it is as violent and unforeseen as an engine stopping in the middle of the sky . . ." (page 19)

www.ingramcontent.com/pod-product-compliance
Lightning Source LLC
Chambersburg PA
CBHW032124020426
42334CB00016B/1064